A CONC
OF GAST

The Author

M. J. S. LANGMAN
M.D.(Lond.), B.Sc., M.R.C.P.
*Professor of Therapeutics,
City Hospital, Nottingham*

A Concise Textbook of Gastroenterology

M. J. S. LANGMAN

CHURCHILL LIVINGSTONE
EDINBURGH AND LONDON
1973

© LONGMAN GROUP LIMITED, 1973

All rights reserved. No part of this publication may be reproduced, stored in a retrieval system, or transmitted in any form or by any means, electronic, mechanical, photocopying, recording or otherwise, without the prior permission of the publishers (Churchill Livingstone, Ravelston Terrace, Edinburgh)

ISBN 0 443 01024 2

Filmset by Typesetting Services Ltd., Glasgow
and printed offset by T. & A. Constable,
Hopetoun Street, Edinburgh

PREFACE

This book summarizes knowledge in a rapidly growing field. The text is clinically orientated, assumes some simple basic knowledge, and emphasizes in particular the natural history of disease and the likely outcome of treatment, but fundamental pathophysiological information is not neglected.

A special feature is the inclusion of tables which summarize findings in clinical analyses and therapeutic trials which are typical of general findings. References are given to these, to sources for further general reading, and to recent work which illustrates current trends.

1973   MICHAEL J. S. LANGMAN

CONTENTS

Chapter		Page
1	Oesophageal disorders	1
2	Peptic ulcer	11
3	Haematemesis and melaena	30
4	Pernicious anaemia, gastritis and other gastric disease	34
5	Malabsorption syndromes	39
6	Appendicitis and other small intestinal disorders	55
7	Large bowel disease	63
8	Crohn's disease	73
9	Ulcerative colitis and ischaemic colitis	78
10	Peritoneal disorders	87
11	Gastrointestinal cancer and polyposis	91
12	Infective diarrhoea	106
13	Intestinal parasites	113
14	Jaundice and hepatic function	118
15	Hepatitis	128
16	Cirrhosis and other liver disorders	134
17	Portal hypertension	147
18	Ascites and hepatocellular failure	152
19	Biliary tract disease	159
20	Pancreatic disease	165
21	Commonly used tests of gastrointestinal function	170
	Bibliography	177
	Index	189

Chapter 1

OESOPHAGEAL DISORDERS

DYSPHAGIA

Difficulty and/or pain on swallowing are ominous symptoms which should never be ignored. By taking a careful history it is usually possible to diagnose the likely site and cause of the abnormality.[10]

Table 1 Commoner causes of dysphagia and their clinical features

Oropharynx
Pouch—swelling in neck on swallowing which can be emptied—dysphagia especially with liquids
Tumours—progressive difficulty and pain in the act of swallowing
Web—food sticks as it enters the gullet
Thyroid enlargement—obvious
Senile rumination—inability to transfer solids to the throat
Neuromuscular disorders—coughing and retching on swallowing; signs of the disorder, e.g. fibrillating tongue in progressive muscular atrophy; return of liquids through the nose

Oesophagus
Achalasia, early stages—retrosternal chest pain and difficulty with solids or liquids, relief with trick procedures, e.g. taking iced water; late stages—no or little dysphagia but regurgitation of sour fluids and chest infections
Stricture—non-progressive or only slowly progressive; no problem with liquids but solids occasionally impact
Carcinoma—rapidly progressive, remorseless, initially for solids then also for liquids
Reflux—long history of heartburn, postural symptoms, non-progressive regurgitation of bitter fluids
Oesophageal spasm—painful swallowing and pain in the chest at other times, often mistaken for cardiac pain

Questioning and examination should be structured to distinguish lesions of the oropharynx from those of the gullet itself and to assess the rate of progression of the lesion. Table 1 lists some of the commoner abnormalities and some of their distinguishing features.

PHARYNGEAL POUCH

Pathology

This, the commonest variety of pharyngo-oesophageal diverticulum, tends to occur in men more often than women. Its cause is uncertain but it probably arises secondary to a rise in pharyngeal pressure due to inco-ordination or spasm of the cricopharyngeal sphincter.

Clinical features

Symptoms and signs include regurgitation of food, often on bending or lying down, dysphagia for fluids rather than solids, and occasionally the patient notices a neck swelling.

Diagnosis and treatment

Barium swallow examination including lateral films is diagnostic. Treatment is by surgical excision of the pouch and sphincter section.[9]

OTHER DIVERTICULA OF THE OESOPHAGUS

Mid or lower oesophageal diverticula can develop as a result of distortion due to juxta-oesophageal inflammatory disease, or can occur just proximal to the hiatus as epiphrenic diverticula. They are usually found incidentally and seldom cause symptoms: treatment (if needed) is by excision.

HIATUS HERNIA AND OESOPHAGITIS

Hiatal herniae can be divided into three common types.
(*a*) Sliding: in which the cardia slides up into the chest, taking its attached ligaments and peritoneal reflexion with it.

(b) *Rolling*: in which a pouch of fundus of the stomach rolls up beside the cardia and into the chest.

(c) *Mixed sliding and rolling hernia*: a combination of both the first two.

All types can become fixed in the chest, or can remain free so that the hernia is only produced by appropriate posturing.

In addition a rare variety of hiatus hernia occurs in association with a congenital short oesophagus.

All types may be associated with oesophageal reflux; but this is in general less common when the gastro-oesophageal junction remains fixed below the diaphragm.

The precise mechanisms preventing reflux are uncertain, but the following have been emphasized.[10]

(a) Physiological cardiac sphincter. Manometric pressure studies have clearly demonstrated the presence of a sphincter zone at the bottom of the gullet which is sensitive to a variety of stimuli, for instance contracting harder in response to a rise in intra-abdominal pressure. This sphincter zone has been found to be less active in those with symptomatic oesophageal reflux, and has recently been considered to be of greater rather than, as formerly, lesser importance.

(b) Mucosal flap valve. There is evidence suggesting that the lower oesophageal mucosa normally projects slightly into the stomach and thus forms an inert flap valve.

(c) Size and activity of the diaphragmatic pinch cock. The right crus of the diaphragm normally compresses the lower end of the gullet from side to side and alters the angle at which it enters the stomach.

Clinical features

The symptoms of hiatus hernia and oesophageal reflux are most conveniently considered together, for they are interrelated in a complex fashion.[13] Hiatus hernia commonly occurs without any symptoms whatsoever, particularly in elderly people with almost total gastric herniae, where herniae may be seen incidentally on chest X-ray.

By contrast there may be no demonstrable hernia but severe symptoms and easily demonstrable oesophageal reflux.

The classical symptoms associated with reflux are retrosternal burning pain together with regurgitation of bitter fluid, worse after meals and on bending and lying down and relieved by alkalis. Active oesophagitis is frequently associated with retrosternal soreness after swallowing. It is well nigh impossible to distinguish symptoms due to hernia alone, though this lesion may give rise to vague discomfort and distension after meals.

Complications

(a) Stricture. Patients with active oesophagitis may develop a fibrosing stricture: usually in association with an oesophageal ulcer.

(b) Anaemia. Iron deficiency anaemia due to slow chronic blood loss is common with hiatal herniae: but it is unwise to attribute acute blood loss simply to a hernia.

(c) Ulcer. (1) Lower oesophageal ulcer is particularly likely to develop in patients who have small areas of ectopic gastric epithelium in the gullet. (2) Simple chronic gastric ulcer occasionally develops at the level of the diaphragm in the mucosa of a hernia.

Assessment

The ability of radiologists to demonstrate herniae or reflux varies considerably and it is always wise to consider carefully before attributing symptoms to these apparent abnormalities. Assessment of the importance of reflux can be aided by oesophagoscopic observation of active inflammation and by carrying out an oesophageal acid perfusion test with N/10 HCl.[12] A good correlation can usually be found between symptoms and their provocation by acid.

Treatment

Most patients with herniae or reflux respond symptomatically to simple medical measures. These include: (a) weight reduction in the obese, (b) small frequent meals, (c) liberal alkali administration, (d) blocking the head of the bed by about six inches at night and also avoiding stooping, (e) oral ferrous sulphate supplements for anaemia.

Those with severe resistant symptoms, strictures, or oesophageal ulcers usually require operative treatment. This should combine repair of the hernia and relief of any stricture with a procedure (such as vagotomy) designed to reduce gastric acid output.

OTHER RARER VARIETIES OF DIAPHRAGMATIC HERNIAE

1. Anterior herniae—usually containing colon—through the foramina of Morgagni: often causing no symptoms.
2. Posterior herniae—containing stomach or colon—through the pleuroperitoneal sinuses (foramina of Bochdalek); this condition can be a cause of respiratory distress in the newborn.
3. Traumatic hernia—usually left sided.

PHRENIC AMPULLA

Barium swallow frequently reveals a small pouch lying above the cardia which does not contain gastric mucosal folds. The appearances, which are a normal pattern on oesophageal distension by a bolus, are often mistaken for a true hernia.

ACUTE OESOPHAGITIS

Apart from inflammation due to reflux of acidic gastric contents or, after gastric surgery, of alkaline duodenal juice containing bile, oesophagitis may be caused by corrosive poisons and by infections.

(a) Due to the ingestion of corrosive poisons, e.g. sodium hydroxide. Necrosis may be mucosal or full thickness leading to mediastinitis. Oral feeding should cease immediately (and gastrostomy may be necessary). Infections need treatment with broad spectrum antibiotics. Steroid therapy may perhaps delay or prevent the later development of stricture but the evidence is unconvincing. Once strictures have developed, they may require dilatation or resection with colonic replacement.

(b) In association with tuberculosis, syphilis (tertiary disease), fungus infections (e.g. monilia), and cytomegalovirus infections. Appropriate specific treatment is available for the first three of these.

OESOPHAGEAL STRICTURE

Strictures arise as a consequence of inflammatory damage due to reflux, to the swallowing of corrosives and following radiotherapy of the gullet. Dysphagia due to stricture is usually only slowly progressive and for solids rather than liquids.

Treatment

Fibrotic strictures due to corrosives and radiotherapy need cautious dilatation at oesophagoscopy. The treatment of stricture associated with reflux is considered on page 4.

OESOPHAGEAL WEB

Patients—usually female—with severe chronic iron deficiency, may develop diffuse epithelial changes such as glossitis and atrophic gastritis as well as anaemia and koilonychia. If there are oesophageal changes they take the form of a thin fibrous web in the upper gullet. This is usually seen on simple barium swallow or with cine radiology. It has also recently been suggested that oesophageal webs can develop independent of any iron deficiency.

Prognosis

Ferrous sulphate supplements and oesophagoscopic destruction of the web are required.

Treatment

The condition does not tend to recur, provided iron deficiency is rectified, but there is an increased liability to postcricoid carcinoma.

EXTRINSIC OESOPHAGEAL DISEASE

Dysphagia may be due occasionally to:
(a) Extrinsic pressure from enlarged hilar glands, for instance secondary to bronchial carcinoma, or from an aortic aneurysm.
(b) Gastric carcinoma infiltrating the cardia.

(c) Aberrant right subclavian artery passing behind the oesophagus (dysphagia lusoria). If symptoms are severe, then the artery should be divided.

DISORDERS OF MOTILITY

Achalasia of the cardia

Pathology

There is a general disturbance of oesophageal motility with loss of the normal peristaltic wave (due to degeneration of intramural ganglion cells) and failure of the cardia to relax on the arrival of a food bolus. The cause is unknown.

Clinical features

Early stages. Features include pain which is retrosternal in site, worse on taking food; liable to relapses and remissions and associated with sticking of food (solid and liquid) in the gullet and occasional prompt regurgitation of the undigested food together with ropes of sticky oesophageal mucus and swallowed saliva. The dysphagia may be relieved by taking a cold or fizzy drink or by the Valsalva manoeuvre.

Late stages. Dysphagia tends to remit and be replaced by dull retrosternal discomfort and regurgitation of sour fluid on stooping and lying down, even long after meals.

Diagnosis

Early stages. There may be no dilatation and barium sulphate may appear to pass (by gravity) easily into the stomach or only be held up slightly. Bread soaked in barium may, however, be held up and an antigravity swallow will show inability to push the contrast medium uphill. The absence of a peristaltic wave can be confirmed, for completeness rather than necessity, by manometric studies with miniature balloons placed sequentially in the gullet. Diffuse motor disorder can also be demonstrated by hypersensitivity to mecholyl. (A classical physiological response to denervation.)

Late stages. Gross oesophageal dilation is obvious (often even on chest X-ray) and there is much retained food residue in the gullet. The lower end of the oesophagus shows a smooth conical narrowing and the gastric air bubble is lost—due to the oesophageal water seal.

Complications

(a) Pulmonary spillover disease. Recurrent pneumonia and bronchiectasis are late complications of gross stasis.
(b) Carcinoma of the midoesophagus. Presumably due to chronic irritation in a stagnant gullet.

Treatment

Bouginage has been discarded as ineffective. Medical treatment with glyceryl trinitrate, and amyl or octyl nitrite may give temporary relief of symptoms but the only logical measures are forcible dilatation of the cardia or Heller's procedure (oesophageal cardiomyotomy).

Dilatation with a pneumatic or metal dilator is designed to rupture muscle fibres but not the mucosa: it is not a procedure for the occasional performer.

Heller's operation is the preferred procedure[11] giving good results in most hands, provided that gross dilatation has not occurred—though even then it is worth attempting. The length of the gastro-oesophageal incision must be sufficient to split the cardia properly, but if overextensive, may predispose to oesophageal reflux.

OESOPHAGEAL SPASM

Diffuse oesophageal muscular spasm, a condition in which there are irregular contractile (tertiary) waves, is an uncommon condition of unknown cause. The associated retrosternal discomfort may mimic that of cardiac infarction, though there is usually a relationship to eating. Barium swallow reveals the characteristic corkscrew appearance due to the irregular tertiary contractions.

Treatment

Anticholinergic drugs such as propantheline may be helpful in relieving pain.

Prognosis

In some patients there is progression to achalasia of the cardia, but in many the condition remains static.

CHAGAS' DISEASE OF THE OESOPHAGUS

Infection with *Trypanosoma cruzei*, a relatively common disease in Brazil and other areas of South America, is followed in some individuals by abnormalities of the gut and heart. The gastrointestinal changes are due to degeneration of the intramural nerve plexus, presumably directly consequent upon the parasitic disease. The oesophageal changes mimic those of achalasia of the cardia (and treatment is similar). Elsewhere the disease produces megaduodenum and megacolon by an identical pathological process.

PROGRESSIVE SYSTEMIC SCLEROSIS (SCLERODERMA)

Dysphagia is a common complication of this generalized connective tissue disease. It is due to loss of the peristaltic wave as the gullet musculature becomes progressively infiltrated by fibrous tissue.

Treatment

Corticosteroids and para-aminobenzoate have been recommended, but there is no good evidence to support their use.

OESOPHAGEAL ATRESIA

Pathology

This congenital anomaly is found in one in every 3000 live births. The main varieties are: (a) with distal tracheo-oesophageal fistula (the majority), (b) without any tracheal fistula, (c) with proximal and distal tracheo-oesophageal fistula, (d) with proximal tracheo-oesophageal fistula only.

It should be suspected in infants of low birth weight or in pregnancy complicated by hydramnios (because this is often associated with upper intestinal obstruction). Other anomalies (commonly duodenal and anorectal malformations) are found in up to a half of the cases.

Clinical features

Respiratory distress after birth due to inhaled secretions manifests itself by episodes of cyanosis and choking, made worse by feeding.

Diagnosis

An oesophageal tube passed through the mouth will be stopped at about 10 cm. The diagnosis can be confirmed radiologically be showing the site of arrest of a radio-opaque tube. If air is detected in the intestine, then the condition must be complicated by a distal fistula re-communicating between the lower oesophagus and the bronchial tree.

Treatment

Immediate management includes nursing prone, which reduces lung spillover, aspiration of secretions and administration of oxygen (below 40 per cent concentration because of the risk of retrolental fibroplasia at higher concentrations). Control of hypoglycaemia with intravenous dextrose, and hypothermia by warming may also be needed. Surgery is based upon division of fistulae and anastomosis of the two blind ends of the gullet but other procedures may be needed, such as gastrostomy and delayed closure (in poor risk infants) or reconstruction with a colonic graft (where the atretic segment is long).

Chapter 2

PEPTIC ULCER

Peptic ulcers are, by definition, found in close association with areas where acid and pepsin secretion occur. Ulcers may be acute or chronic and occur in the lower oesophagus, stomach, duodenum, jejunum or in association with a Meckel's diverticulum.
Pathophysiology. Peptic ulcer is assumed to be due to an imbalance between the erosive action of the secretions and the strength of mucosal resistance, but knowledge of the more precise causes of ulceration is poor.

Acute ulcers

These are usually small, often multiple, evanescent, shallow, epithelial breaches with little or no fibrous reaction. They do not seem to be associated with excessive acid output, indeed bleeding acute gastric ulcers often seem to be associated with relative hypochlorhydria and some degree of atrophic gastritis, suggesting that poor resistance rather than powerful corrosion may be important.

Chronic gastric and duodenal ulcers

Site. Duodenal ulcers tend to occur in the first or occasionally second part of the duodenum. Gastric ulcers are usually found on the lesser curve or posterior wall of the stomach, especially at the junction of the pyloric and parietal mucosa. Ulcers also often occur on the superior antral wall: they are rarely found on the greater curve, except in patients who have been taking antirheumatoid drugs such as phenylbutazone. Chronicity of ulceration is indicated by penetration of the muscularis mucosae (and often deeper muscle coats) and by the fibrous scarring reaction to ulceration.

Acid output. Chronic duodenal ulcer tends to be associated with a large parietal cell mass demonstrable by acid hypersecretion in response to stimulation with pentagastrin, and with a relatively low intragastric pH in the resting stomach, even though total acid output at this time is not excessive. There is, however, a considerable overlap between the acid secretory powers of the stomach in normal people and in those with duodenal ulcers. By contrast, acid output tends to be normal or even reduced in patients with gastric ulcer.[15]

Mucosa. Apart from an increased parietal cell population, the gastric mucosa is histologically normal in duodenal ulcer. By contrast, in gastric ulcer the non-parietal mucosal area is usually increased, especially on the lesser curve and there is often some degree of histologically demonstrable gastritis.[23] Biliary reflux through the pylorus is also a common finding in patients with gastric ulcers and it has been suggested that the combination of bile and acid may be particularly damaging to the mucosa, possibly by causing back diffusion of hydrogen ions into it and thus disrupting intracellular organelles.[14]

Aetiology

Acute ulcers. Associations have been noted with burns (Curling's ulcer), mid-brain disease (Cushing's ulcer) and with debilitating disease in general. Aspirin containing analgesics may also induce acute ulcer bleeding, though the risk of this complication has been overstated.

Chronic peptic ulcers. There is much epidemiological evidence which suggests that the incidence and behaviour of peptic ulcers varies according to the site at which they occur and, therefore they should not be considered as a single entity.[6]

Temporal trends and sex ratio

Gastric ulcer was common in most areas of Western Europe, especially in young women, until the end of the 19th Century, but since then duodenal ulcer, which formerly seems to have been rare, became the predominant variety and its incidence rose steadily initially in men and later in women and probably reached a maximum about ten years ago, since when its incidence seems to have declined a little. The present picture in Western Europe of duodenal ulcer is of a disease which is three times commoner in men than in women with a peak frequency at the age of 30 to 50 years. By contrast, gastric ulcer tends to be found more often with advancing age and to be only slightly more frequent in men than in women. This pattern is not constant, however, and there are marked geographical variations throughout the world.[6]

Occupation

Both gastric and duodenal ulcer (especially the former) tend to be commoner amongst the unskilled and semiskilled and their families than in those in professional and administrative occupations.

Diet, smoking and alcohol

Though diet is likely to be of special importance, no single factor has convincingly been shown to influence ulcer incidence and there is no evidence that mild to moderate alcohol consumption is associated with an increase in ulcer incidence. Ulcers have, however, been found more frequently in smokers than in non-smokers.

Genetics

There is a distinct familial and genetic influence upon ulcer incidence. Both duodenal and gastric ulcers, especially when complicated by bleeding, are more common in individuals of group O than in those of groups A, B and AB, and they are more common in general in those who are constitutionally incapable of producing these blood group substances in their mucous secretions (non-secretors).

Mucosal surfaces are rich sources of blood group substances, but no proof has yet been obtained that these influence acid secretion or act as direct mucosal defences.

Drug-induced ulcer

Antirheumatoid drugs such as phenylbutazone and corticosteroids almost certainly exacerbate ulcer symptoms, but it is hard to prove that they cause ulcers to develop *de novo*.

Excessive aspirin based analgesic intake has been suggested as an important cause of chronic gastric ulcer which is frequently found in young women in Australia,[24] though curiously the same problem does not seem to occur elsewhere, despite the enormous amounts of salicylates consumed annually.

Other varieties of peptic ulcer

Oesophageal ulcer. Reflux of acid and pepsin into the gullet can cause discrete areas of ulceration as well as diffuse oesophagitis, and this is discussed elsewhere.

Zollinger-Ellison syndrome. A rare but distinct variety of fulminating ulceration, often in the lower duodenum or upper jejunum has been found to be associated with an enormously increased acid output by the resting stomach. Patients with the condition have grossly raised serum gastrin concentrations in association with pancreatic hyperplasia, adenomatosis or carcinoma of γ or gastrin producing cells. They also often have other endocrine tumours or have relatives with such tumours, for instance in the parathyroid glands.

Postoperative ulcer. Recurrent duodenal, or occasionally gastric ulcer and, if gastroenterostomy has been performed, gastrojejunal ulcer, are well known sequelae to gastric surgery; they have the same pathological features as other varieties of ulcer.

Clinical features

Pain. Peptic ulceration is classically associated with intermittent upper, usually midline, abdominal pain which is relieved or aggravated by food and which occurs in bouts of weeks or months interspersed with equivalent periods of freedom from symptoms. Though the pain of duodenal ulcer is frequently worse two or three hours after food or at night, whereas gastric ulcer pain is often more closely related to meals, the clinical characteristics of ulcer pain are such poor discriminants that no reliance can be placed upon them. Pain going through to the back suggests, however, that the posterior gastric wall (an area difficult to see on X-ray or at gastroscopy) or post-bulbar duodenum may be the site of ulceration.

Vomiting. Vomiting of large quantities of fluid containing old food residues strongly suggests the presence of pyloric obstruction whilst iron deficiency anaemia is a well known occasional concomitant of duodenal or (usually large) gastric ulcers.

Haemorrhage and perforation. Approximately a fifth of gastric or duodenal ulcers in men, and rather less in women, cause acute haemorrhage or perforation and these are often the presenting features of the disease. Occasionally ulcers, especially if large, can cause iron deficiency anaemia—often as a presenting feature.

Physical signs. Physical examination tends to be unhelpful diagnostically except in demonstrating anaemia, or the succussion splash or visible peristalsis of pyloric obstruction. The presence or absence of epigastric tenderness has no special clinical significance.

Diagnosis

Radiology of gastric ulcer

Lesser curve ulcers. Barium meal examination is by far the most important diagnostic measure. A lesser curve chronic ulcer is usually seen as a distinct niche or pocket of barium projecting out from the line of the barium filled stomach. The crater has a clean smooth outline and often its upper part contains a fluid level between barium below, and gastric juice or gas above. A posterior wall gastric ulcer is often best seen *en face* as a barium filled niche after a small amount of the barium suspension has been drunk and when the abdomen has been compressed. A spastic notch on the greater curve opposite the ulcer is a common feature of chronic gastric ulcer. Occasionally a gross horizontal fibrous contracture in association with longstanding ulceration can cause a permanent hour glass constriction, or the lesser curve can shorten longitudinally.

Antral ulcers and malignancy. Antral or prepyloric ulcers present special diagnostic difficulties to the radiologist because the associated spasm or inflammatory swelling cannot always be distinguished from the appearances of gastric cancer. Greater curve ulceration is uncommon except in patients taking antirheumatoid drugs and is seldom malignant (despite previous contrary views). Lesser curve ulcers above the angulus can usually be separated with confidence from malignant disease by their regularity and relative absence of mucosal distortion within the line of the barium filled viscus (except by the classical appearances of fibrous contracture). The size of gastric ulcer is not a guide to the presence of malignancy nor to the severity of symptoms; furthermore large gastric ulcers often respond better to medical treatment than small ulcers.

Radiology of duodenal ulcer. The radiological diagnosis of duodenal ulcer is bedevilled by the problem of distinguishing simple deformity in the duodenal cap, due to previous and now healed ulceration from deformity with active ulceration.

Ulceration in an undeformed cap is relatively uncommon. It may be seen either as a niche in profile on one border of the cap, or *en face* through the cap when it contains a small quantity of barium suspension and is either compressed, or else air contrast films are obtained, such as in a posterior view with the patient lying slightly on his left side. Scarring of the cap can induce a number of deformities such as trefoil deformity following ulceration at the base of the cap, and pseudo-diverticulum formation.

A minority of ulcers occur in the immediate postbulbar region of the duodenum, and close attention to this area is needed if these are to be found.

Endoscopy

Modern fibreoptic instruments have greatly increased the safety, diagnostic range and comfort for the patient, of endoscopic examination. The available instruments are either end or side viewing. The former are good general purpose instruments which allow an adequate view of the oesophagus, of the stomach and the upper duodenum, whereas side viewing instruments tend to be more specialized, and present models give good views of the lesser curve of the stomach (less well seen with end viewing instruments). The newer small diameter varieties are particularly useful in duodenal examination.[18]

The main use of gastroscopy lies in the separation of benign from malignant ulceration in cases where the distinction cannot be made with certainty by radiology. Simple ulcers appear as regular punched out defects in the mucosa, containing a greyish-white slough. Malignant lesions may appear more irregular, and the surrounding mucosa is often frankly nodular in contradistinction to the simple oedema in the region around a benign ulcer. Biopsy should be done routinely.

Endoscopy can also be a useful primary diagnostic tool in patients where barium meal examination has been normal despite a typical ulcer history.

Gastric function tests in ulcer diagnosis

Patients with duodenal ulcer tend to have a relatively large parietal cell mass and can, therefore, secrete somewhat increased amounts of acid gastric juice, whereas those with gastric ulcers—particularly on the lesser curve—tend to have a reduced, or normal, acid secretory capacity. However, the overlap between the normal and the ulcer range is so great, even in duodenal ulcer, that there is a lack of discriminating power upon which diagnostic confidence can be placed.[15]

Gastric analysis does, however, have a limited usefulness in that a high rate of stimulated secretion combined with a low basal output can suggest, though not confirm, the presence of a duodenal ulcer in a dyspeptic patient with a normal X-ray. By contrast anacidity following stimulation with pentagastrin or histamine in a patient with gastric ulcer is a strong indication that the lesion is malignant. Furthermore, a comparison of basal and maximal stimulated acid secretory activity is one of the principal methods by which the Zollinger-Ellison syndrome can be distinguished. Most individuals with the condition will have a high rate of stimulated secretion but also a basal unstimulated secretory rate which is at least 40 per cent of the stimulated output.

Serum pepsinogen determination. This is no more useful in ulcer diagnosis than direct acid measurements.

Plasma gastrin determination

The evidence so far available suggests that plasma gastrin concentrations are not diagnostically different in normal people and in patients with gastric or duodenal ulcer. Unusually high levels (as might be expected) are found in the Zollinger-Ellison syndrome, and in pernicious anaemia (because of the loss of acid inhibition of gastrin release by the antrum).[16,17]

Management of Peptic Ulcer

Medical treatment of simple uncomplicated ulcer

The basic aims of treatment are to relieve symptoms, to heal the ulcer and to prevent relapse or complications. In practice, however, there is no proven method of preventing relapse or the occurrence of complications. Radiological assessment offers a simple and reasonably reliable method of measuring gastric ulcer healing, but the problems of differentiating between scarring and active ulceration make this well nigh impossible in duodenal ulcer, except in the uncommon patients with craters but without deformity. The success of duodenal ulcer treatment must therefore be largely judged by symptomatic response.

Gastric ulcer, relief of symptoms

Ulcer pain, as in duodenal ulcer, is usually relieved by simple measures including alkali administration, bed rest and small frequent meals. This is considered in detail in the section on duodenal ulcer.

Acceleration of gastric ulcer healing

Traditional treatment of proven value

Bed rest in hospital and stopping smoking have both been clearly shown in well conducted clinical trials to accelerate healing (Table 2).

Sedation, dietary treatment, intensive alkali, and milk and alkali treatments have not been shown to have any significant effect upon ulcer healing, despite their value in symptom relief.

Newer treatments

Carbenoxolone sodium. This substance, a triterpene with structural resemblances to corticosteroids, though not itself a steroid, is synthesized from glycyrrhizinic acid extracted from liquorice root, which has long been a folk remedy for dyspepsia.

Table 2 Effect of treatment on gastric ulcer healing

	Average reduction in size of ulcer niche(%)	No. of patients
Bed rest (inpatients 4 weeks)[20]	59	32
Ambulant (outpatients)	15	32
Advised to stop smoking[19]	78	40
Not advised to stop smoking	57	40
Carbenoxolone 300 mg daily for 4 weeks[21]	72	30
Dummy tablets	35	20
Carbenoxolone 300 mg daily for 1 week, then 150 mg daily for 4 weeks[22]	70	19
Dummy tablets	46	17

Table 2 shows that when treatment with carbenoxolone is given to ambulant out-patients the results are at least equivalent to those obtained by traditional means. However, complications of salt and water retention often occur, especially in the elderly and with increasing doses of the drug, as sometimes do hypokalaemia and raised blood pressure. To reduce the frequency and severity of these complications it is wise to prescribe less than 150 mg daily of the drug to patients over 65 years of age, and to avoid it in all those with significant cardiorespiratory or renal disease.

During treatment patients should be seen weekly and their weight and blood pressure checked. Unexpected weight gain, in excess of 4 lb (2·0 kg) is an indication for concurrent diuretic treatment. Spironolactone should be avoided because it prevents ulcer healing as well as fluid retention;[25] thiazide diuretics together with a potassium supplement such as Slow K (because of the risks of hypokalaemia with simultaneous carbenoxolone and thiazide treatment) are usually effective.

Good evidence that continued carbenoxolone treatment in small doses will prevent relapse has yet to be obtained, but relapse following treatment seems to be no more frequent than after other conventional therapy.

The mode of action of the drug is unknown; it is completely absorbed in the stomach and does not affect acid secretion; it is therefore assumed to increase mucosal resistance.

Deglycyrrhizinated liquorice: this is a preparation of crude liquorice root from which most of the glycyrrhizinic acid, from which carbenoxolone is synthesized, has been removed. Controlled trial experience is considerably less than that obtained with carbenoxolone, but it seems to be largely free of side effects, except mild diarrhoea. In the one trial of sufficient size to make comparisons worthwhile, results roughly equivalent to those reported with carbenoxolone have been obtained.[26]

Other treatments

1. Oestrogens. These appear to be ineffective.
2. Gefarnate. This is the geranyl ester of farnesyl acetic acid and is claimed to be of value in treating gastric ulcer, but the results of substantial controlled comparisons are not yet available.
3. Antipepsins. A small controlled trial carried out in the U.S.A. suggests that a synthetic sulphated mucopolysaccharide (Depepsen) will accelerate gastric ulcer healing. This finding needs confirmation.[27]

Duodenal ulcer

Bed rest and diet

Though ulcer symptoms usually settle rapidly during bed rest there is no good evidence that this response is matched by ulcer healing or affects the final outcome of the disease.

The use of diets based upon milk and milk products is hallowed by tradition, but has never been proved to be of clinical value. Recent evidence in fact suggests that such foods have no more effect upon gastric acidity than freely chosen diets.[31,32]

Small frequent meals may, however, be useful because their neutralizing effect will prevent marked swings of gastric acidity. Patients are also often advised to reduce their alcohol, coffee and tea consumption and to stop smoking. These measures seem sensible and often seem to help individual patients, though they have never been proved to be of general value.

Antacids

The effect upon gastric acidity of the small doses of alkali usually prescribed in clinical practice is much more short-lived than the relief obtained from symptoms. Aluminium and magnesium based preparations, such as aluminium hydroxide and magnesium trisilicate, and sodium bicarbonate are effective, cheap and free of side effects in conventional doses (apart from occasional constipation with aluminium and diarrhoea with magnesium salts). Large doses cause more prominent side effects and have yet to be shown to be of greater value. Calcium carbonate should not be used for, though a potent antacid, it can cause hypercalcaemia and even small rises in serum calcium concencentrations have been found to be associated with 'rebound' acid hypersecretion (thus possibly explaining the association between duodenal ulcer and hyperparathyroidism).[29]

Anticholinergics

These drugs, such as propantheline, poldine and glycopyrrolate, can be justified theoretically on the grounds that they will reduce gastric acid output. Some results also suggest that ulcer symptoms and relapse rates are also reduced. There is also an equal body of findings which suggests that these drugs have no detectable effect.[28,30] Despite the fact that (unlike atropine) they are supposed to have a selective action on the stomach, they still can cause dry mouth, urinary retention and aggravate glaucoma. They should also never be used in patients with pyloric obstruction because they will reduce gastric antral pumping activity.

Carbenoxolone capsules

Possibly because they are absorbed completely in the stomach, carbenoxolone tablets seem to be ineffective in duodenal ulcer. Timed release capsules have therefore been designed with the object of delivering their contents direct into the duodenum. Conflicting results have been obtained with this preparation.[33]

Deglycyrrhizinated liquorice and gefarnate

The former, after initial promising findings, has ultimately been found to be ineffective in duodenal ulcer[34,35] and the latter has yet to be properly tested.

Oestrogens

Though stilboestrol was initially shown to be useful in duodenal ulcer in men, side effects of mastitis and impotence have been too common to permit its routine use.

Gastric irradiation

Radiation will alleviate ulcer symptoms by producing temporary necrosis of gastric parietal cells. However, the long term risks of leukaemia and perhaps cancer are such that the treatment can virtually only be used in those with intractable symptoms but in whom surgery is inadvisable because of poor general health.

Management of Complications

Haematemesis and melaena. These are considered in Chapter 3.

Perforation

Diagnosis

The sudden onset of severe pain, associated with marked abdominal rebound tenderness, loss of bowel sounds and the presence of free gas under the diaphragm on straight X-ray clearly denote free perforation of a hollow viscus. Confusion can occasionally occur with acute pancreatitis or cholecystitis when bowel sounds will likewise sometimes be lost (though there will not be free gas demonstrable).

Misdiagnoses of acute abdominal conditions requiring laparotomy are of little or no importance, but more serious confusion, for instance with coronary thrombosis or pneumonia, is well known.

Treatment

(a) By operation: morphine is given as soon as possible to relieve pain and the patient is prepared for operation, the remaining stomach contents being removed through a gastric tube. Simple suture is the quickest and easiest procedure, but patients with long clinical histories and who are in good general condition are often treated by a definitive surgical procedure such as vagotomy and pyloroplasty, because the chances of recurrent symptoms would otherwise be high.

(b) Conservative management: aspiration of gastric contents and maintaining the empty stomach thereafter for 48–72 hours will lead to spontaneous closure of the leak by fibrinous exudate. In experienced and enthusiastic hands, this method gives equivalent results to suture and in the gravely ill patient may be the only possible procedure, but early operation is the best method for general use.

Prognosis

Short term mortality is affected in particular by: 1. the interval between perforation and start of treatment; 2. the type of ulcer present, acute or chronic; 3. the patient's age.

Pyloric stenosis

Clinical features

This is commonly due to duodenal ulceration though it can arise with prepyloric ulceration or gastric cancer. A chronic peptic ulcer history prior to obstruction is usual, the symptoms of pain being replaced by vomiting, often of large volumes, typically containing old food residues, and a succussion splash is easily elicited.

Progression to the late stages is associated with marked dehydration, weight loss and the development of visible gastric peristalsis. Electrolyte disturbances are common and the loss of hydrogen ion and of sodium, chloride and potassium leads to a combination of low serum sodium and high bicarbonate. The alkalosis is emphasized by potassium depletion affecting renal function, conservation of hydrogen ion being impaired and leading to paradoxical aciduria. Tetany with positive Trousseau's or Chvostek's signs due to the alkalosis is uncommon but well recognized.

Treatment

This includes: (a) correction of fluid and electrolyte imbalance by intravenous infusion of saline with a potassium chloride supplement; (b) removal of stagnating gastric contents with a large bore gastric tube.

Anticholinergic drugs should be avoided because they will reduce gastric antral motility, and antacids in large quantities will make the electrolyte disturbance worse.

Pylorospasm: The sudden onset of obstructive symptoms in patients with active ulcers may only be due to pylorospasm and will usually respond to simple conservative measures.

Organic stenosis: Once fluid and electrolyte balance have been regained and any other features such as anaemia corrected, then operation should be carried out, a drainage procedure such as gastroenterostomy being combined (except sometimes in the very elderly) with a measure (such as vagotomy) to prevent ulcer recurrence.

Elective Surgery for Peptic Ulcer

Indications

There are as yet no clear predictive features which will allow one to judge which patients will ultimately need operation because of continued symptoms or complications and which will not. The primary indications for operation therefore remain as severe acute or recurrent bleeding, perforation, cicatrization and obstruction, and prolonged symptoms inadequately relieved by medical treatment.

Operations

All procedures commonly performed, apart from simple suture of a perforation, are designed to reduce acid secretion and may be combined with ulcer excision and a drainage procedure.

Gastric ulcer

Simple ulcer excision is rapidly followed by recurrence, and the choice at present lies between partial gastrectomy with gastroduodenal anastomosis (Billroth I) and vagotomy plus pyloroplasty.[36,37]

Billroth I gastrectomy usually gives good results associated with a low mortality (approximately 1 per cent) and few post gastrectomy problems. Vagotomy plus drainage is also usually effective; the mortality may be slightly less but there are more indications that this less well tried procedure gives a much higher recurrence rate, especially in lesser curve ulceration (Table 3).

Table 3 Clinical results of two gastric ulcer operations[37]

Percentage of patients with:	Billroth I gastrectomy	Vagotomy with pyloroplasty
Good overall clinical result	88	66
Recurrent ulcer	2	14

Duodenal ulcer

The large number of operations which have been devised is a measure to some extent of the dissatisfaction with available measures.

Simple gastroenterostomy. Postoperative stomal ulcer recurrence is so common that this procedure has no place except perhaps in the very elderly with simple pyloric obstruction.

Billroth I partial gastrectomy with gastroduodenal anastomosis. This operation has been discarded because of the high postoperative recurrence rate.

Polya or Billroth II partial gastrectomy with gastroenterostomy. Following disillusionment with Billroth I gastrectomy, this became the most popular definitive procedure for duodenal ulcer. Recurrent stomal (or rarely gastric) ulcer is uncommon, but its disadvantages include a raised mortality rate, a high incidence of symptomatic disorders such as bilious vomiting and dumping, and an increased incidence of anaemia and (probably late metabolic complications).

Vagotomy and drainage procedures. Dissatisfaction with Polya gastrectomy has led to the widespread acceptance of vagotomy, to reduce acid output, plus drainage by pyloroplasty, gastroenterostomy or with antral excision, to prevent postvagotomy gastric retention. However, vagotomy has been found to be associated with complications, notably of diarrhoea and raised recurrent ulcer incidence due to incomplete nerve section as demonstrated by postoperative insulin testing.

Comparative results and postoperative problems

Table 4 illustrates some of the clinical results which have been obtained in Leeds and York during a comparison of four commonly performed ulcer operations.[38] The overall findings indicate that approximately three quarters of operations give satisfactory clinical results, but illustrate in particular the problems of dumping with procedures including an enterostomy and diarrhoea with vagotomies.

Table 4 Clinical results of duodenal ulcer operations[38]

Percentage of patients with:	Operation			Polya partial gastrectomy
	Vagotomy plus			
	Gastroenterostomy	Antectomy	Pyloroplasty	
Bile vomiting	15	14	10	13
Diarrhoea	26	23	22	7
Dumping	24	13	12	22
Proven or likely recurrent ulcer	6	2	11	2
Overall result perfect or only mild occasional symptoms (included above)	70	78	68	77

Recurrent ulcer. (i) After Polya gastrectomy, this is usually simply cured by vagotomy. (ii) After vagotomy, re-operation and section of the remaining nerve fibres is usually satisfactory, though partial gastrectomy may be required.

Dumping. A complex of symptoms of nausea, sweating, palpitations, faintness, and abdominal fullness develops, usually after gastroenterostomy, and it is probably due to overfast meal emptying into the jejunum followed by a rapid output of fluid into the lumen with gut distension.

Treatment: Simple measures such as small, frequent meals with a low fluid and carbohydrate content are often sufficient. Medical treatments with insulin and tolbutamide (because of supposed endocrine disturbance by rapid carbohydrate absorption) are usually unhelpful. Surgery with conversion to a Billroth I (gastroduodenal) anastomosis may be required.

Vomiting. This may be due to organic obstruction by a recurrent ulcer or narrow pyloroplasty. It may also commonly be due to biliary regurgitation and consequent gastric irritation.

Treatment: Medical treatment is unsatisfactory, though metoclopramide may help (dose 10 mg three times daily), and Roux en Y anastomosis may be required.

Diarrhoea. This is primarily a postvagotomy complication with watery bowel motions and much urgency, or occasionally steatorrhoea (cause unknown). However, surgery can unmask latent lactase deficiency or gluten enteropathy, and rapid emptying through a gastroenterostomy stoma can cause functional pancreatic insufficiency due to poor mixing. Diarrhoea may also rarely be due to recurrent ulceration and the formation of a gastro-jejuno-colic fistula.

Treatment: The frequency of postvagotomy diarrhoea has led to the development of selective gastric vagotomy and comparative results suggest that diarrhoea may be less when gastric vagal branches only are cut.

Postvagotomy diarrhoea tends to improve slowly and gradually with time but responds poorly to drug treatment. Codeine phosphate 30 mg three or four times daily may be helpful. Trial of milk withdrawal or even gluten withdrawal may also occasionally be worthwhile.

Selective and superselective vagotomy

Though resection of gastric vagal branches may be followed by a reduced incidence of diarrhoea it is as yet unclear whether the operation is more or even less effective than standard vagotomy in curing duodenal ulceration.[39]

A natural development has been superselective (parietal cell only) vagotomy in the hope of avoiding the drainage procedure needed in the remaining varieties of operation because of the gastric retention which otherwise occurs. This procedure is still in the stages of preliminary assessment.

Metabolic Consequences of Gastric Surgery

In the succeeding years after gastric surgery occasional patients develop complications of anaemia, bone disease and steatorrhea. These vary in frequency according to the operation undertaken, but become more common after ten or more years have elapsed.[40,41]

Polya gastrectomy

Anaemia. This is usually mild and of iron deficiency type and is due to a combination of inadequate intake and poor absorption of iron. More rarely megaloblastic anaemia occurs secondary to intrinsic factor deficiency or, occasionally, to competition for vitamin B_{12} by bacteria contaminating a blind loop.

Treatment: Iron deficiency responds well to oral or parenteral iron. Ferrous sulphate tablets 300 mg once or twice daily are usually perfectly adequate. Yearly haemoglobin measurement and prompt treatment of mild deficiency is a wise precaution.

Vitamin B_{12} deficiency demands standard pernicious anaemia treatment with hydroxocobalamin (Chapter 4).

Bone disease

Osteomalacic bone disease is an uncommon late complication, often, but not always associated with steatorrhoea. It should be suspected in patients with complaints of muscular weakness (bone pain usually develops late). The diagnosis is confirmed by a low serum calcium and high alkaline phosphatase (in the absence of liver disease or Paget's disease). Loosers zones (pseudofractures) may be seen radiologically, especially in the pubic rami, ribs and scapulae. Bone biopsy to show widened osteoid seams, may be necessary in some patients.

Treatment: Calcium and vitamin D supplements are needed. In prescribing these it should be remembered that the calcium content of different supplements varies widely, as does the vitamin D content of standard preparations, see Table 5. The latter is especially important because the distinction between the toxic and the therapeutic dose of vitamin D is very small. Strong calciferol tablets should therefore only be prescribed for patients with clear evidence of malabsorption or where the smaller dietary supplement present in calcium with vitamin D is ineffective. Response to treatment should be checked by reference to changes in serum calcium and alkaline phosphatase concentrations.

Table 5 Calcium and vitamin D supplements

Calcium content of standard therapeutic preparations	Calcium content per gram (approx.)
Calcium lactate	120 mg
gluconate	80 mg
carbonate	360 mg
Milk	125 mg/100 ml
Vitamin D content of standard therapeutic preparations	
Calcium with vitamin D B.N.F.	12·5 μg per tablet
Strong calciferol	1·25 mg

Steatorrhoea. This complication is due usually to poor mixing and rapid emptying of the stomach and upper bowel: occasionally pancreatic deficiency is the cause. It is often helped by pancreatic supplements (Chapter 5).

Billroth gastrectomy with gastroduodenal anastomosis. Metabolic complications are infrequent and consist mainly of occasional iron deficiency anaemia (poor intake with restricted stomach size) and, more rarely, vitamin B_{12} deficiency (due to resection of intrinsic factor secreting cells and to gastric atrophy). Bone disease and steatorrhoea are uncommon. Treatment is the same as for Polya gastrectomy complications.

Vagotomy and drainage. Anaemia, steatorrhoea and bone disease are probably less frequent than after procedures including gastric resection but follow up experience is, as yet, inadequate for any confident conclusions to be possible.

Radiologically negative abdominal pain. The majority of people who have barium meals or cholecystograms because of abdominal pain prove to have normal X-rays. It should be remembered that such pain may arise from musculoskeletal disorders, for instance referred from the spine, from the genitourinary tract, or simply be an expression of underlying anxiety or depression. Less commonly pain is due to neurological disorders, such as *Herpes zoster*, tertiary syphilis and epidemic myalgia, may be thoracic in origin or a symptom of constitutional or endocrine disorders such as porphyria, polyarteritis, familial Mediterranean fever, haemochromatosis, Addison's disease and lead poisoning.

Chapter 3

HAEMATEMESIS AND MELAENA

Aetiology and epidemiology

More than three quarters of all episodes of haematemesis and melaena in the United Kingdom are caused by peptic ulceration; individual causes and their frequency are given in Table 6.

Table 6 Causes of acute upper gastrointestinal bleeding, Central Middlesex Hospital, London (1941–1965)[1]

Peptic ulcer group	Percentage
Chronic gastric ulcer	16·6
Chronic duodenal ulcer	34·6
Acute lesions/X-ray negative	26·7
Postoperative	6·3
Hiatus hernia	2·3
Unclassified	3·1
Non-ulcer group	
Gastric cancer	2·5
Portal hypertension	2·7
Others*[44]	5·2

*Simple tumours e.g. leiomyoma; hereditary telangiectasia; haemorrhagic states; haemophilia, von Willebrand's disease; thrombocytopenia; Peutz Jeghers syndrome; cancer of oesophagus and pancreas; Mallory Weiss syndrome (oesophageal mucosal tear).

Drug-induced bleeding and peptic ulcer

Many patients, particularly those with acute erosions give a history of aspirin intake in the two to three days before admission. It is also well known that unbuffered salicylate preparations cause superficial gastric mucosal damage and occult micro-bleeding in most people. However, the problem of 'salicylate induced' bleeding is more complex than these simple facts would suggest. Thus there is a gross disparity between the enormous amounts of aspirin consumed in the United Kingdom and the low incidence of acute bleeding. In addition those with 'salicylate induced' haematemesis or melaena seem to be no more sensitive on re-exposure to these compounds than control individuals. Salicylates seem likely to be no more than a minor contributing factor to the incidence of acute upper gastrointestinal bleeding.[42]

Liver disease and haemorrhage

Though oesophageal varices are an expected by-product of raised portal pressure in hepatic cirrhosis, bleeding in cirrhotics is at least as commonly due to coincident peptic ulceration as to a ruptured varix. The management of varices is considered in detail on page 147.

Management of Bleeding

All patients with recent (within 48 hours) acute blood loss of more than minimal quantity should be admitted to hospital.

Blood replacement

This is the single vital measure, but the need may be difficult to judge because, especially in the young, the classical clinical features of pallor, sweating, tachycardia and low blood pressure may be absent. In addition it must be remembered that recent blood loss will not have resulted in anaemia because there will have been insufficient time for haemodilution to occur.

As a broad guide transfusion is needed if: (a) the initial haemoglobin concentration is less than 10 g per cent; (b) there are classical clinical features of shock—not due to complicating pancreatitis or ulcer perforation; (c) blood loss is visibly or by reliable accounts substantial.

In elderly patients and those with cardiovascular disease, circulatory overload can be prevented more easily if the infusion cannula is passed into the superior vena cava so that any undue rise in central venous pressure can be monitored.

Bed rest and diet

Although bed rest, a light diet and liberal fluid intake are sensible initial measures, there are no grounds for enforcing rest or withholding a normal diet after the first few days.

Sedation

Though this may help to calm anxious patients, it is doubtful if 'routine' sedative treatment has any virtue.

Investigation

Early barium meal investigation and/or fibreoptic endoscopy are frequently recommended and will undoubtedly increase the precision of diagnosis. In areas (such as the U.S.A.) where oesophageal varices are relatively common as a cause of bleeding, early diagnosis may alter management, but in other areas (such as the United Kingdom) where ulcer bleeding is by far the commonest cause, it is uncertain if it makes a significant contribution.[43] There is as yet no convincing evidence that intensive early investigation will lead to a lowered mortality from haematemesis and melaena.

Length of stay in hospital

Ulcer bleeding is unlikely to recur (in the short term) when 4 days have elapsed since admission and it is certainly safe to discharge patients 10 days after admission with uncomplicated bleeding.

Recurrent haemorrhage and indications for operation

Elderly patients (and those with recurrent bleeding) are particularly likely to die (Table 7). Surgery must therefore be considered carefully in these. The type of ulcer present probably does not materially affect the decision to operate, though a long dyspeptic history and a proven chronic ulcer—especially gastric —weight the scales in favour of surgery.

At operation a careful search must be made to ensure detection of the bleeding lesion, and a long gastrotomy may be required to allow adequate examination of the stomach in locating acute erosions which are often multiple and sometimes high in the stomach.

Table 7 Influence of age on outcome with haematemesis and melaena (Radcliffe Infirmary, Oxford 1953–1967)[45]

Age	Total number of patients	Deaths (%)
<40	331	2·7
40–59	798	4·8
60–79	852	13·5
80+	168	17·9

Acute lesions often demand no more than under-running of the bleeding vessel, but chronic ulcers need definitive surgery. Billroth I gastrectomy is still the standard procedure for gastric ulcer, but duodenal ulcer is increasingly being treated by the technically simpler vagotomy and drainage procedures rather than by Polya gastrectomy. Gastrectomy has given good results in the past in the United Kingdom, though curiously not in the U.S.A. (Table 8) but the long term results of vagotomy and drainage are as yet unclear.

Table 8 Late recurrence rate following admission with bleeding duodenal ulcer

		Follow up (years)	Relapse rate (%)
Great Britain[46]	Medical treatment	5–10	20
	Surgical treatment	5–10	2
U.S.A.[47]	Medical treatment	5	44
	Surgical treatment	5	18

Chapter 4

PERNICIOUS ANAEMIA, GASTRITIS AND OTHER GASTRIC DISEASE

The ability to produce acid and intrinsic factor are lost together in patients with gastric atrophy. However, vitamin B_{12} deficiency leading to pernicious anaemia or, much more rarely, subacute combined degeneration of the spinal cord takes several years to supervene because of the large liver stores of the vitamin.

Pathophysiology

In the complete atrophy of pernicious anaemia, gastric glandular and all parietal cells are lost, and the mucosa is infiltrated by large numbers of plasma cells and lymphocytes. Immunofluorescent studies will demonstrate antibodies to intrinsic factor and to parietal cells in serum, secretions and mucosa in most patients. Though the presence of such antibodies is a useful pointer, they are not diagnostic because they can, for instance, be demonstrated occasionally (and parietal cell antibodies frequently) in patients with simple atrophic or chronic superficial gastritis without vitamin B_{12} malabsorption.

Aetiology

The cause of pernicious anaemia is not understood. The presence of auto-antibodies, mucosal infiltration by plasma cells and reversibility of the gastric lesion by corticosteroids suggest an auto-immune process. There is also a small but definite genetic predisposition, the disease being, like gastric cancer, slightly more common in individuals of group A than in those of the remaining ABO groups.

Diagnosis

(a) Pentagastrin. The gastric pH will remain greater than 6·5 after the injection of pentagastrin 6 µg/kg intramuscularly or ametazole (Histalog) a histamine analogue. Indirect testing by urine collection following an oral dose of Azure A (theoretically, absorbed in the presence of acid only) yields too many false positive results to be useful.

(b) Serum vitamin B_{12}—measured by bacterial (e.g. *Strep. faecalis*) or isotopic assay, less than 70 picograms/ml—but can be similarly low for a considerable time in prepernicious anaemia before liver stores are exhausted.

(c) Schilling or other direct tests of vitamin B_{12} absorption using the radioactively labelled vitamin. A standard pack (Dicopac) containing ^{57}Co and ^{58}Co labelled vitamin B_{12} allows simultaneous testing of absorption with and without intrinsic factor. Normal subjects will excrete at least 7 per cent of an oral dose of labelled vitamin B_{12} in the urine in the 48 hours after ingestion, provided a flushing injection of a large (e.g. 1000 μg) dose has been given simultaneously. If the flushing dose is not given, the labelled preparation, if absorbed, will accumulate in the liver slowly over 7–14 days (forming the basis of the liver uptake test).

(d) Assay of intrinsic factor secretion by (for instance) charcoal immuno-assay.

Treatment

Hydroxocobalamin has replaced cyanocobalamin because it is better retained in the body. A dose of 200 μg by injection every month is more than sufficient to maintain body stores after loading treatment with 1000 μg on three alternate days.

Prognosis

Patients with treated pernicious anaemia have a normal life expectancy apart from a slightly increased risk of gastric cancer. This increase, a three to fourfold multiplication compared with the general population, is still too low to make regular screening for gastric cancer profitable.

Congenital pernicious anaemia

This rare condition, inherited as a Mendelian recessive is due to an inherited inability to secrete intrinsic factor in adequate amounts. It presents as megaloblastic anaemia in infancy and is associated with normal acid secretory potential. The specific failure of intrinsic factor synthesis in this condition must be distinguished from congenital ileal receptor deficiency for the vitamin B_{12}—intrinsic factor complex (Imerslund's disease) and from vitamin B_{12} deficiency due to gastric failure in the hypoparathyroidism candidosis syndrome.[180]

Gastritis

This term is better used to describe specific histological abnormalities of the gastric mucosa rather than (as is frequently done) to describe dyspeptic symptoms in those who have no demonstrable ulcer.

Chronic superficial gastritis

In this condition inflammatory cells infiltrate the superficial mucosa but gastric glands are well preserved. It has been found with increased frequency in those who smoke excessively or who consume large amounts of alcohol or hot beverages.[48] No specific symptom pattern has been correlated with it, and it does not seem necessarily to predispose to gastric atrophy.

Chronic atrophic gastritis

In addition to cellular infiltration there is a loss of gastric glands, and acid and pepsin secretory capacity is reduced in parallel. It does not cause symptoms but in a minority of patients there is progression to the complete atrophy of pernicious anaemia. Patients with atrophic gastritis probably also have a similar liability to the later development of gastric cancer to those with pernicious anaemia.

Giant hypertrophic gastritis

Giant mucosal rugal hypertrophy occurs in association with the Zollinger-Ellison syndrome and rarely as an isolated entity (Menetrier's disease). In the latter condition gastric acid output is usually reduced but there is excessive secretion of protein (see Protein losing enteropathy, Chapter 5). Subtotal gastrectomy may be required to control the protein loss.

INFANTILE PYLORIC STENOSIS

Pathology

In this condition the muscle of the pyloric canal is unduly hypertrophied, the cause being unknown. It is much commoner in boys than girls (sex ratio approximately 5:1) is a frequent anomaly (incidence about 3 per 1000 live births) and is thought to be due to a combination of genetic predisposition and some abnormality of foetal or early postnatal development.

Clinical features

Symptoms usually develop in the first few weeks after birth and characteristically consist of copious projectile vomiting of the gastric contents after feeding. On examination there is usually visible gastric peristalsis and a lump can be felt abdominally in the region of the pylorus. Barium meal examination is not usually necessary but will confirm the presence of a 1–2 cm long narrow segment at the pylorus. The condition must be distinguished principally from oesophageal atresia (onset at birth and difficulties with swallowing) and duodenal obstruction/atresia (bile stained vomit).

Treatment

A minor proportion of all cases settle in the first two to three months with conservative management with anticholinergic drugs, and atropine methonitrate is often used, though it is doubtful if it confers any special advantages. Most will require Rammstedt's procedure (pyloromyotomy) and early surgery is in general preferable to prolonged medical management.

ADULT HYPERTROPHIC PYLORIC STENOSIS

Occasional adult patients present with obstructive symptoms due to pyloric stenosis associated with muscular hypertrophy. Rarely this is due to recurrence of infantile pyloric stenosis; it is usually associated with juxtapyloric peptic ulceration, but sometimes the problem seems to be due to primary hypertrophic stenosis arising in adult life.

Treatment. Pyloric obstruction requires pyloroplasty together with a procedure such as vagotomy if there is an associated juxtapyloric ulcer.

PYLORIC MUCOSAL DIAPHRAGM

This rare condition which probably represents an incomplete form of duodenal atresia, can present with obstructive symptoms like those of pyloric stenosis in childhood or adult life. Treatment is surgical.

GASTRIC DIVERTICULA

These occur most commonly near the cardia on the lesser curve, but occasionally are found in the prepyloric region. They seldom cause symptoms and their principal importance lies in the likelihood of confusion with gastric ulceration.

VOLVULUS

Partial (antral) or total gastric volvulus are rare causes of acute upper abdominal pain and vomiting. They can arise *de novo*, or as torsion within a hiatus hernia.

Treatment. Gastric aspiration is followed by surgical relief of the volvulus.

ACUTE DILATION OF THE STOMACH

Pathology. Sudden gross gastric distension can arise after any form of upper abdominal surgery, including cholecystectomy and especially after vagotomy, after childbirth and in diabetic coma. The causes are uncertain.

Clinical features and treatment. Vomiting of relatively clear gastric contents is succeeded by the production of dirty brown or faeculent material and the development of abdominal distension. Prompt decompression with a large bore stomach tube and intravenous fluid replacement are required.

Chapter 5

MALABSORPTION SYNDROMES

Malabsorption syndromes occur in a large variety of diseases which interfere with the absorption of nutrients.[49] Diarrhoea is not always a symptom and patients can present with vague abdominal complaints or nutritional deficiencies. Investigation for evidence of poor absorption should always be considered in patients with nutritional deficiencies without obvious cause.

The approach to the patient should be structured in three parts: (a) demonstrating malabsorption (Chapter 21); (b) assessing specific deficiencies (Table 9); (c) defining the cause[50,51] (Table 10).

Table 9 Clinical features of malabsorption

Deficiency	Clinical problem
Total calorie	Weight loss and wasting
Protein	Oedema (uncommon)+muscle wasting
Fat	Weight loss
Iron, vit. B_{12}, folate	Anaemia, glossitis and stomatitis
Vit. D, calcium, magnesium	Bone pain, muscular weakness, tetany
Vit. K	Spontaneous bruising, purpura
Multiple vitamin and calorie	Depression, neuropathy, short stature, amenorrhoea, infertility

Clinical features

Diarrhoea.[52] Steatorrhoeic stools are classically described as pale, unformed, malodorous, greasy and difficult to flush away, whilst in carbohydrate diarrhoea, they tend to be watery and frothy due to the presence of fermented sugars. Rectal bleeding is uncommon—unless there is a coagulation defect due to vitamin K deficiency.

Abdominal symptoms. Flatulent non-specific distension and discomfort are extremely common presenting features, but severe pain is rare except in pancreatitis or carcinoma, and occasionally in inflammatory bowel disease.

Nutritional disturbances. Tiredness, glossitis, anaemia, bone pain (due to osteomalacia) and weight loss are common and can be related to specific deficiencies (Table 9).

PANCREATIC DEFICIENCY

Fat and protein are malabsorbed as also may be vitamin B_{12} (though this rarely causes clinical problems). Steatorrhoea is common but anaemia and bone disease are relatively infrequent.

Diagnosis

Pancreatic steatorrhoea may be differentiated from other varieties by the Lundh and secretin—pancreozymin tests (Chapter 21). In chronic pancreatitis calcification may be visible on a plain radiograph, the glucose tolerance curve may be diabetic and hypotonic duodenography may show abnormal folds. Fibrocystic disease can be diagnosed by assessment of faecal tryptic activity and, most elegantly, by determining sweat sodium and chloride concentrations after skin iontophoresis of pilocarpine (chloride concentration usually greater than 70 mEq/litre in the disease).

Treatment

A low fat and high protein diet are usually effective. Pancreatic supplements have to be given in large doses and tend to be unpleasant. Nutrizym (a preparation containing vegetable proteases as well as pancreatic extracts) one tablet with meals may have advantages over conventional treatment with Pancrex V forte 3–4 tablets with each main meal.

BILE SALT DEFICIENCY SYNDROMES

Pathophysiology

Bile salts are actively conserved by the body being re-absorbed in the terminal ileum and colon, and resecreted approximately ten times each day (Fig. 1). To be effective in promoting fat absorption they must be present as conjugates, and in sufficiently high concentration to promote mixed micelle formation. Steatorrhoea due to bile salt deficiency is seldom severe because long

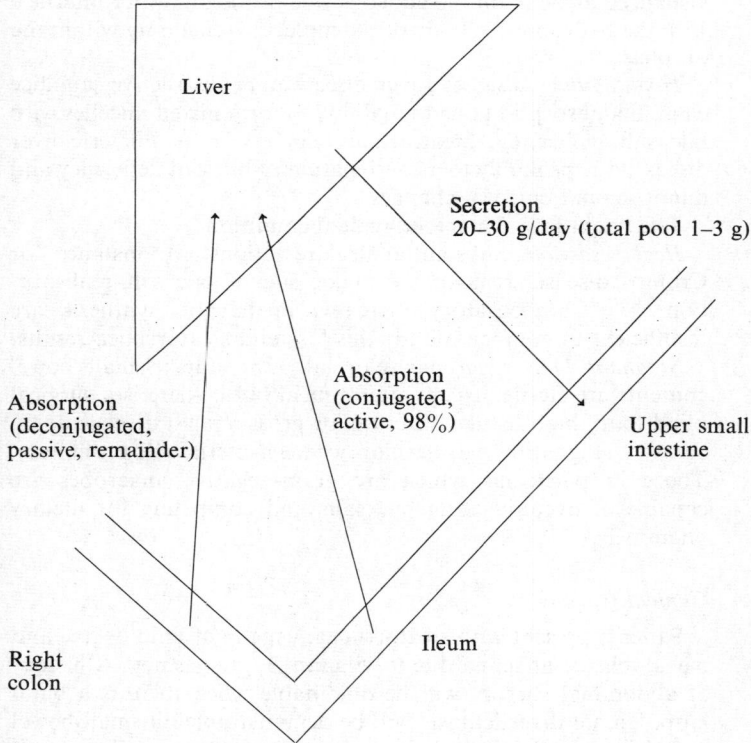

Fig. 1 Bile salts. Enterohepatic circulation and properties.[53]

Bile salts: glycine and taurine conjugates of bile acids, pK 4 and 2 respectively therefore always ionized at pH 5. Critical concentrations required for formation of mixed micelles approximately 4 mmol. Bile acids: cholic (trihydroxy) and chenodeoxycholic (dihydroxy), bacteria convert these to desoxycholic (dihydroxy) and lithocholic acids respectively. pK of bile acids > 6, therefore relatively ineffective in promoting mixed micelle formation.

chain monoglycerides and fatty acids, the products of triglyceride hydrolysis by pancreatic lipase, can to some extent be absorbed from non-micellar mixtures. By contrast cholesterol and (probably) fat soluble vitamin absorption are heavily dependent upon mixed micelle formation. In these structures the bile salts lipophobic hydroxy and polar (ionic) groups can be visualized as lying on the aqueous side of the oil–water interface with the hydrophobic body of the molecule remaining within the oil phase.

Hepatobiliary disease. Liver disease and obstructive jaundice cause malabsorption due to inability to form mixed micelles with bile salt deficiency. Steatorrhoea can occur in anicteric liver disease, due probably to a combination of bile salt deficiency and minor jejunal mucosal changes.

Treatment is as for the individual condition.

Ileal resection. Substantial ileal resections, for instance for Crohn's disease, remove the major site of bile salt reabsorption.[55,57] Compensatory increases in hepatic synthesis are insufficient to compensate for this loss and steatorrhoea results.

Stagnant loop syndrome. Normally the upper small bowel contents are sterile, except after a meal but if there is a surgical blind loop, high fistula, stricture, or gross jejunal diverticulosis, areas of stagnation can develop where bacteria will proliferate. Those in particular which are gram-negative anaerobes are capable of deconjugating bile salts and competing for dietary vitamin B_{12}.[56]

Clinical features

Patients present with steatorrhoea, usually of mild degree and megaloblastic anaemia due to vitamin B_{12} deficiency. A history of abdominal surgery will be obtainable when there is a blind loop, jejunal diverticulosis will be demonstrable on small bowel radiology and fistula by follow through or (more easily) enema examination. Vitamin B_{12} malabsorption will not be correctable by intrinsic factor administration, and sampling studies will demonstrate high concentrations (greater than 10^8 per ml) of bacteria including anaerobic *Bacteroides*, and *E. coli*.[54]

Treatment

Fistulae, strictures and blind loops should be removed surgically. Bacterial contamination of diffuse jejunal diverticulosis can usually be controlled by antibiotics such as tetracycline 250 mg two or three times daily.

COELIAC DISEASE

This, the commonest form of steatorrhoea,[61] can present at any stage from early childhood to late adult life. It is caused by small intestinal sensitivity to a protein fraction of wheat gluten which induces villous stunting, though intestinal cellular turnover is increased rather than decreased.

The mechanism is unknown and peptidase deficiency and (more likely) an immunological abnormality have been suggested.[58] The latter is supported by evidence of increased cellular immunological activity in the small bowel wall and by the frequent finding of antireticulin (antibasement membrane) antibodies in the serum.[59] The disease tends to occur in families more often than would be expected by chance.

Clinical features

Childhood. Failure to thrive on a mixed diet, diarrhoea and anaemia—usually of iron deficiency type—are common problems.

Adults. Steatorrhoea does not always occur, and many adults present with megaloblastic (folate deficient) anaemia and bone pain due to osteomalacia. Further investigation may reveal multiple (usually fat soluble) vitamin deficiencies, iron deficiency and sometimes minor degrees of vitamin B_{12} deficiency. Splenic atrophy, with the presence of Howell Jolly bodies in the blood is common.

Diagnosis

Xylose excretion is grossly reduced (Chapter 21), and steatorrhoea is usually but not always demonstrable chemically (faecal fat excretion at least 18 g over a 3-day period on a good mixed diet) but the critical procedure is jejunal biopsy. Histology and dissecting microscopy reveal varying degrees of villous stunting or complete villous loss giving a flat mucosa with abnormal flattening of epithelial cells and inflammatory cellular infiltration of the villous stroma. The changes are maximal in the upper jejunum, and are not entirely specific to coeliac disease for similar, but usually less severe changes have been found in association with ulcerative colitis, Crohn's disease and carcinomatosis and tropical sprue, amongst others.

Treatment

Almost all childhood cases, and most adults respond to a gluten free diet. However, if there are only isolated deficiencies— such as folate deficiency—simple dietary supplementation may be adequate. Severe cases may initially need dietary supplements of folic acid, calcium and vitamin D together with a gluten-free diet.

Response is associated with a return of xylose[60] and fat excretion and haematological abnormalities, as well as intestinal biopsy appearance towards normal. Simple constipating drugs such as codein phosphate (30 mg two or three times daily) are useful in ameliorating troublesome diarrhoea in the early stages.

Complications: failure to respond to diet

(a) Inadequate appreciation of the scope and desirability of dietary restriction. This is the commonest cause of failed response.
(b) Secondary milk (lactose) intolerance[63] (see p. 51).
(c) Intestinal lymphoma.[62] There is now good evidence that patients with long standing or recently diagnosed coeliac disease may develop intestinal reticulosis or lymphoma.
(d) Idiopathic failure. Persistent problems sometimes respond to treatment with prednisone 10 mg three or four times daily, but a few show no improvement, and some have been shown to have collagen deposits below the mucosa (collagenous sprue).[64]

Other complications and associated disease

Peripheral neuropathy, sideroblastic anaemia, fibrosing alveolitis,[65] intestinal perforation and haemorrhage and a variety of skin changes have been described in association with coeliac disease. Dermatitis herpetiformis is frequently associated with malabsorption[66] and intestinal mucosal changes typical of coeliac disease, but usually of milder degree.[67]

TROPICAL SPRUE

Pathology

This condition[68] affects the small intestine equally throughout its length. The histological abnormalities of villous stunting are like, but less severe than, those of coeliac disease. The cause is unknown, but it is especially frequent in some tropical areas such as southern India and Puerto Rico. This patchy distribution together with response to antibiotic treatment suggests an infective cause.[69]

Clinical features and diagnosis

Diarrhoea, usually steatorrhoeic in type, is common and there are associated non-specific abdominal symptoms, glossitis, weight loss and later, anaemia.

Malabsorption with onset in the tropics should always suggest this diagnosis. The association of mild small intestinal biopsy abnormalities with vitamin B_{12} malabsorption, uncorrectable with intrinsic factor confirms it.

Treatment

Megaloblastic anaemia, if present, usually requires treatment for combined vitamin B_{12} and folate deficiency. These haematinics together with broad spectrum antibiotics, such as tetracycline, usually produce prompt initial improvement. However, the precise effects of treatment, at least in Europeans, are hard to judge, because natural remission usually occurs on leaving endemic areas.[70] A few individuals have persistent problems even in temperate climates and may require a high protein low fat diet with vitamin supplements and antibiotics.

CROHN'S DISEASE

Malabsorption may be due to bile salt deficiency consequent on ileal abnormalities, fistulae, large resections and blind loops. It is discussed in Chapter 8.

INFILTRATIVE DISEASE

Amyloid disease and progressive systemic sclerosis both can cause steatorrhoea by interfering with function by submucosal infiltration.

The former is usually demonstrable by rectal biopsy and the latter is usually associated with characteristic skin changes. Lymphoma is often associated with coeliac disease.

WHIPPLE'S DISEASE

Pathology

In this condition the small intestine mucosa, lymph glands and often other tissues such as pericardium, heart, pleura and meninges contain large numbers of abnormally foamy cells which stain with periodic acid Schiff (P.A.S.). The cause is uncertain but the response to antibiotics, and electron microscopic changes suggesting the presence of bacteria in the mucosa strongly suggest an infective basis.

Clinical features

Diarrhoea and steatorrhoea are commonly associated with generally enlarged lymph glands, arthropathy, a raised E.S.R., fever and skin pigmentation. Less often patients have pericarditis, pleural and meningeal involvement.

Diagnosis

Intestinal mucosal or lymph gland biopsy will reveal the characteristic P.A.S. staining of macrophages and the abnormally blunted leaf shaped villi. Rectal biopsy may also be diagnostic.

Treatment

Prolonged (18–24 months) treatment with either tetracycline or ampicillin in full doses will cure the condition.

RESECTION AND BYPASS

Malabsorption may be due either to the effects of removal of extensive lengths of small bowel (for instance with repeated operations for Crohn's disease), to stagnation and bacterial contamination, inadvertent gastro-ileal bypass and to rapid emptying after Polya gastrectomy. The problems of stagnant loops and postgastrectomy diarrhoea are discussed on pages 27 and 28. Distal resections will remove the areas absorbing bile salts and vitamin B_{12}: these functions cannot be taken over by the jejunum but the ileum can undertake iron and folate absorption after jejunal resections.

Massive resections are followed by remarkably little metabolic upset until only a few feet of small intestine remain.

Treatment

Patients with distal resections giving vitamin B_{12} malabsorption require conventional vitamin B_{12} treatment as for pernicious anaemia.

After massive resections patients may have especial difficulty in absorbing long chain fats. Replacement of these in the diet by medium chain triglyceride (M.C.T.) a mixture of ten carbon atom average fatty acid chain length, supplies a water miscible fat which is readily absorbed and transported in the portal venous blood. In addition patients need a high protein diet with appropriate vitamin supplements.

IRRADIATION AND VASCULAR INSUFFICIENCY

The former can give rise to diffuse fibrous tissue infiltration and to stricture formation, whilst the latter can impair small intestinal function—often causing intestinal angina—without causing ischaemic necrosis.

Lymphatic obstruction

Any disease (see Table 10) interfering with lymphatic drainage can cause fat malabsorption. Congenital lymphangiectasia, a disease in which lymphatic drainage channels have failed to develop properly, responds moderately well to dietary replacement of long chain fats with medium chain triglyceride. Intestinal biopsy reveals the characteristic distended lymphatics in the villi.

Table 10 Causes of malabsorption

Pancreatic deficiency	Inflammation
	Carcinoma
	Fibrocystic disease
Bile salt deficiency	Liver and biliary disease
	Ileal resection
	Stagnant loop syndrome—blind loops, strictures and fistula, diverticula
Loss of functional absorptive surface	
Direct mucosal damage	Coeliac disease
	Tropical sprue
	Inflammation—Crohn's disease
	Infiltration—amyloid, scleroderma, lymphoma
	Whipple's disease
Surgery: resection and by-pass	
Irradiation	
Vascular insufficiency	
Lymphatic obstruction	Congenital lymphangiectasia, retroperitoneal fibrosis, heart disease, lymphoma
Infections	Tuberculosis, *Gardia lamblia*, strongyloidiasis, hookworm
Endocrine	Thyrotoxicosis, diabetes mellitus, Zollinger Ellison syndrome
Drugs	PAS, neomycin, phenindione, cholestyramine
Biochemical abnormalities	Disaccharidase deficiency
	Monosaccharide malabsorption
	Abetalipoproteinaemia
	Enterokinase deficiency, tryptophan and methionine deficiencies
Immunological	Pernicious anaemia, agammaglobulinaemia, alphachain disease

Infections

Tuberculosis is a rare cause of malabsorption, and steatorrhoea has been recorded in association with strongyloidiasis, hookworm and giardia infections. The tape worm, *Diphyllobothrium latum* also competes preferentially for vitamin B_{12}. Treatment is discussed in Chapter 13.

Endocrine disturbances

Thyrotoxicosis is sometimes associated with mild steatorrhoea, and intestinal stagnation consequent upon neuropathy may be the cause of steatorrhoea seen occasionally in diabetics with apparently normal pancreatic exocrine function. The steatorrhoea of Zollinger-Ellison syndrome is almost certainly due to inactivation of pancreatic enzymes by the large quantity of acid entering the duodenojejunal area.

Drugs

Steatorrhoea due to phenindione and paraminosalicylic acid intake disappears rapidly when the drugs are stopped. In these conditions the cellular anatomy is normal, but neomycin induces temporary partial villous atrophy. Cholestyramine, a bile acid binding resin used in treatment of the pruritus of incompletely obstructive jaundice and in controlling post-hemicolectomy diarrhoea will also cause steatorrhoea if given in sufficiently large doses.

SUGAR MALABSORPTION

Pathophysiology[71]

The sequences and sites of carbohydrate digestion are shown in Figure 2. Abnormalities of most of these processes have been observed clinically and the varieties are summarized in the lower part of the figure. Maldigestion of starch has not proved to be a problem, and sucrase deficiency is not as common in general as lactase deficiency.

Clinical features

Childhood. Infants present with the primary disorder in the neonatal period with failure to thrive, dehydration and watery, frequent, frothy stools. Secondary sugar (usually lactose) malabsorption should be suspected if there is failure to recover from another illness, such as coeliac disease, which stresses the bowel, despite apparently adequate treatment.

Adults. Primary sugar malabsorption. Watery diarrhoea is the usual complaint together with distension, pain and borborygmi, and this complex may be mistaken for a simple irritable bowel syndrome. The diarrhoea is due to the bulk purgative effect of

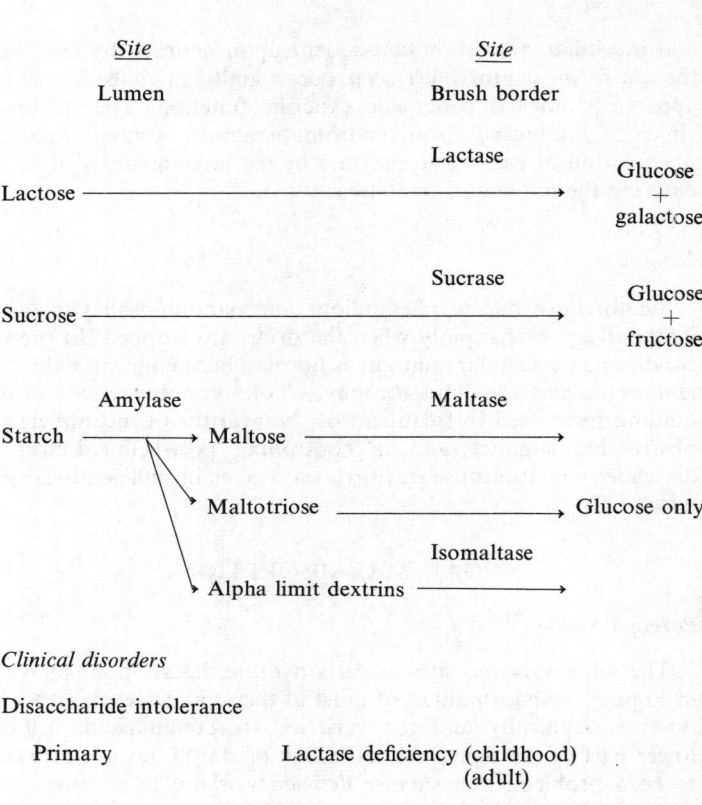

Fig. 2 Sugar absorption and malabsorption

unabsorbed sugars acting as an osmotic load. Frothy acid stools are produced because colonic bacteria break down the sugars to lactic and other acids. Many patients with lactase deficiency will say, if questioned specifically, that they have noticed that milk tends to upset them. The primary condition shows a pronounced racial variation in frequency, being especially common in some African and South European populations.[72] Secondary deficiency manifests itself with other intestinal conditions (as in childhood).

Diagnosis

1. Stool pH. Frothy acid stools with a pH less than 5·5 should lead to suspicion of the diagnosis. In childhood the finding of ½ per cent or more of reducing substances in stools with Clinitest tablets is strongly suggestive.[73]
2. Sugar tolerance tests with lactose or sucrose and their constituent sugars. Patients usually have flat curves and notice exacerbations of their symptoms with the offending disaccharide but not its constituent monosaccharides (see Chapter 21).
3. Diagnostic withdrawal.
4. Assay of disaccharidase activity in mucosal biopsy specimens.

In general a convincing response to sugar withdrawal is an adequate diagnostic manoeuvre in childhood. Sugar loading tests become more practicable in adult life and usually give reasonably accurate and sufficient information (see Chapter 21 for details).

Treatment

Withdrawal of milk sugar or sucrose either permanently in primary disaccharide intolerance or temporarily in secondary intolerance are all that is required.

GLUCOSE–GALACTOSE MALABSORPTION

In early infancy glucose–galactose malabsorption is a rare cause of watery diarrhoea with failure to thrive. It is due to inadequate active transport of these hexoses. The condition is temporary and can be treated by fructose substitution (this sugar is handled by an independent transport system) as in galactomin 19 (Trufood).

ABETALIPOPROTEINAEMIA

This rare generalized condition consists of acantholytic red cells, absent betalipoproteins in the blood and steatorrhoea. The last defect seems to be due to inability to clear absorbed triglycerides.

IMMUNOLOGICAL ABNORMALITIES

Pernicious anaemia—this is considered elsewhere.

Agammaglobulinaemia. There is a protective immunological system for the gut and lungs based upon the secretion of a variety of IgA linked as a dimer with a specific protein (secretory piece) and upon the presence of a large number of immunologically competent cells, mainly producing IgA, in the gut.

Immune deficiencies of this system usually lead to watery diarrhoea and recurrent infections but intractable malabsorption has been described and also arises in alpha chain disease and lymphoma.[74,75]

Alpha chain disease. There is suppression of normal IgM and IgG production locally in the gut and only alpha chains of IgA are produced. Antimitotic drugs may be helpful in treatment.

Lymphoma. This is discussed in relation to coeliac disease.

PROTEIN MALABSORPTION

In general protein malabsorption is not a cause of severe special problems though absorption depends upon specific hydrolysis and active transport systems.

Enterokinase deficiency. This very rare congenital disorder presents in childhood with severe diarrhoea and failure to thrive.

Transport defects. Defects of transport for (a) neutral amino acids (Hartnup disease), (b) dibasic amino acids and cystine (Cystinuria), and (c) glycine, proline and hydroxyproline (Iminoglycinuria). These do not cause gastrointestinal symptoms.

Defects of transport of essential amino acids. There are two very rare varieties, for tryptophan (blue diaper syndrome) and methionine (giving rise to mental defect).

PROTEIN LOSING ENTEROPATHY

Excessive protein loss through the gut wall can occur by exudation, following abdominal lymphatic obstruction, or by excessive secretion perhaps by increased cell turnover. Causes are listed in Table 11, together with methods of measurement. (^{51}Cr) albumen fulfills the necessary criteria for measuring loss as the label is firmly bound to the protein and urinary loss of dissociated isotope is slight. Once the protein is lost into the gut the isotope is excreted quantitatively in the faeces. Protein labelling is simplified by giving ^{51}Cr Cl$_3$ as a direct intravenous injection so that binding to protein occurs *in vivo*. Alternative screening tests, using synthetic macromolecules, employ ^{59}Fe Dextran and ^{131}I Polyvinyl pyrrolidone. ^{131}I labelled protein can be used to estimate rates of synthesis (by examination of blood radioactivity decay curves) but will not give a measure of

Table 11 Protein losing enteropathy

Causes

Exudative protein loss	Cancer of gastrointestinal epithelium, Crohn's disease and ulcerative colitis
Lymphatic obstruction	Primary lymphangiectasia, Whipple's disease, congestive heart failure, lymphoma, retroperitoneal fibrosis
Other causes (secretory loss and rapid turnover)	Coeliac disease, tropical sprue, Menetrier's disease
	Infestations and infections, allergic gastro-enteropathy

Measurement

	Measures Enteric loss	Pool size	Urinary isotope excretion	
(^{51}Cr) Albumen	√	×	√	good standard test
(^{131}I) Polyvinyl pyrrolidone	√	×	√	screening test
(^{59}Fe) Dextran	√	×	×	screening test
(^{131}I) Protein	×	√	√	will measure synthesis in absence of loss

rate of loss as the iodine label when detached from the protein in the gut is re-absorbed and excreted in the urine or resecreted.

ALLERGIC GASTROENTEROPATHY

This rare syndrome usually presents in childhood with diarrhoea and failure to thrive. There is gross oedema due to intestinal protein loss and pronounced circulatory and small intestinal eosinophilia. Allergy to food protein—commonly milk—forms the basis. It responds to appropriate dietary exclusion or (less preferably) to steroid treatment.

Chapter 6

APPENDICITIS AND OTHER SMALL INTESTINAL DISORDERS

ACUTE INFLAMMATION

Pathogenesis

This is a common disease of occidental communities and is presumably dietary in origin but the cause is unknown. Acute appendicitis is often, but not always associated with the presence of obstructing faecoliths, and a mucocoele may develop distally if infection does not supervene upon obstruction.

Clinical features

The classical picture is of central abdominal colicky pain which shifts over several hours to the right iliac fossa and is associated with tenderness, and then rigidity, fever, vomiting and leucocytosis. However, abdominal signs may not be prominent if there is a retrocaecal or ileal appendix, or the organ lies low in the abdomen. Symptoms may then suggest urinary infection and rectal tenderness may be a prominent feature. The classical feature of shifting discomfort is in fact less common than constant right iliac fossa pain.

Treatment

Uncomplicated early disease. Morbidity and mortality rates from acute appendicitis are negligible if the organ is removed before it perforates. Therefore when there are convincing localizing signs, operation should be undertaken promptly in the knowledge that the early removal of a normal appendix will do no harm.[76]

Cases with intermediate signs of acute disease, localized

tenderness, rigidity and an ill-defined suggestion of a mass should likewise be dealt with promptly. Delay gains nothing in that interval appendicectomy will still be required even if the problem settles, and there is a considerable short term risk of general peritonitis.

Late disease. Several hours delay before surgery for resuscitation by fluid replacement, nasogastric suction and antibiotic therapy is clearly correct for the patient with generalized peritonitis due to gangrene, perforation and faecal leakage. Rarely the delay is so great that conservative measures only can be employed.

CHRONIC APPENDICITIS

Chronic, intermittent pain or discomfort in the right iliac fossa is commonly ascribed to chronic appendicitis when no other cause is detectable. However, laparotomy frequently reveals a normal appendix—especially in young women, where the pain is probably of ovarian origin.

Though removal of a high proportion of normal appendices is unjustifiable, the appendix is sometimes abnormal, and symptoms often settle postoperatively. The risk of elective surgery is small and the benefits therefore outweigh the disadvantages if selection is reasonably careful.

OTHER VARIETIES OF INTESTINAL ULCERATION

Peptic ulcer and Meckel's diverticulum

Occasionally Meckel's diverticula contain ectopic gastric epithelium and acute or chronic peptic ulceration can develop with bleeding, occasionally perforation and (not prominently) pain as clinical features. Treatment is surgical.

Primary non-specific and iatrogenic ulcer of the small intestine

This is a rare condition which gives rise to pain, bleeding, stricture and occasionally perforation. The cause is in general unknown except that one variety in which cicatricial narrowing tends to be prominent, is induced by enteric coated potassium chloride tablets. These have therefore been discarded in favour of slow release and effervescent preparations.

SMALL INTESTINAL ISCHAEMIA

Acute infarction

Acute infarction of small bowel may be due to thrombosis or embolism, which usually involves the superior mesenteric artery. Predisposing factors include atrial fibrillation, atheroma, hypotension and intra-abdominal sepsis.

Clinical features. These are of an acute abdominal emergency with shock and peritonitis.

Treatment. Irreversibly damaged bowel must be resected, but sometimes the abnormality is so extensive that no such treatment is possible. Occasionally endarterectomy and embolectomy can be carried out, and would be the treatment of choice for ischaemia which is extensive but looks reversible at operation, and is associated with an accessible proximal block. Conservative treatment with blood and low molecular weight dextran transfusion, and nasogastric suction may be the only possible measures in elderly patients in poor general condition. The results in general are bad, and the value of dextran in particular is doubtful.

Intestinal angina

Abdominal pain with onset after meals, steatorrhoea and weight loss may be due to chronic midgut ischaemia, usually associated with atherosclerosis. For symptoms to develop there must be extensive vascular disease involving at least two of the three main intestinal arteries. Occasionally an abdominal bruit is audible, and poor or absent femoral pulses may suggest the condition, otherwise there are no diagnostic clinical features. Aortography is needed to confirm the diagnosis. Treatment is surgical by endarterectomy or arterial reconstruction.

Acute ileitis and mesenteric adenitis

Occasional patients present with short histories mimicking acute appendicitis but operation shows nothing but acute ileal inflammation or inflamed mesenteric lymph nodes. Such cases settle rapidly and uneventfully with conservative treatment and probably represent responses to viral or other infections, one of which has been characterized as bacterial due to *Yersinia enterocolitica*.[77] Separation is required clinically from Crohn's disease and tuberculous lymphadenitis.

INTESTINAL OBSTRUCTION

Mechanisms. Simple mechanical obstruction at any level is inevitably followed by the proximal accumulation of gas and fluid. Most of the gas particularly in upper intestinal obstruction is swallowed air but lower bowel gas includes significant amounts of methane and carbon dioxide derived from bacterial activity, and also some diffused gas.[78]

In acute obstruction gaseous distension is initially more prominent than fluid distension because at first fluid reabsorption continues unhindered, particularly in loops some distance above the obstruction site. However, as time passes fluid accumulation becomes more obvious because, as the bowel distends, reabsorption becomes less efficient.

Since nearly 20 per cent of the total body water (Table 12) is normally secreted each day, half as salivary and gastric output and half as intestinal and pancreaticobiliary secretion, disturbances of fluid and electrolyte balance soon become obvious due to gross losses by vomiting and into distended loops of gut.

Table 12 Average daily intestinal secretory output (litres) in normal adults

Saliva	1
Gastric juice	3
Bile	1
Pancreatic juice	1
Intestinal secretion	2
	8

Closed loop obstruction

If relief of simple obstruction is delayed then progressive distension, in a peritoneal cavity which is of limited distensibility, will lead to kinking of proximal loops of bowel so that closed obstructed loops develop, which will not decompress when the initial obstruction is relieved. This is especially likely to happen in the colon, where the ileocaecal valve can prevent proximal transmission of distension and lead to colonic perforation.

Functional (pseudo) obstruction

Dilatation of the bowel with accumulation of gas and fluid

can occur in a variety of conditions where there is no mechanical blockage, but bowel function is impaired due to inflammation or metabolic disturbance.

Strangulation and ischaemic obstruction

If a segment of the gut is deprived of its blood supply, for instance by mesenteric arterial thrombosis there is an effective obstruction in the gangrenous segment which will in time perforate. Similar problems can arise if a loop of gut is trapped in a confined space such as a femoral hernia or twists in a volvulus. Initial venous obstruction is followed by tissue oedema and the arterial supply then becomes occluded. These events in their train tend to mucosal ulceration, blood loss into the bowel lumen and perforation.

Clinical features

These will vary according to the level of obstruction and its severity level.
High obstruction. Rapid dehydration occurs due to loss of saliva, gastric and pancreaticobiliary juice but distension is not usually prominent because of the large vomits.
Mid gut (lower ileal) obstruction. Onset of symptoms is usually less acute than with high obstruction and distension will not be prominent because of proximal reabsorption of secreted fluid.
Low (colonic) obstruction. Distension is usually obvious especially with closed loop obstruction, but vomiting is less conspicuous. If allowed to progress perforation of the caecum, or the obstructing lesion itself, may occur.

Severity

Acute obstruction. The condition is rapidly complete and irreversible and there is progressive distension, increase in number of fluid levels on X-ray, and in size of gastric aspirates with general deterioration. Typical causes are colonic cancer and strangulated hernia.
Chronic obstruction. Distension is mild, and there is recurrent colicky pain with fluctuation of bowel habit between constipation and diarrhoea. Inflammatory bowel disease is a typical cause.

Between these two patterns can be found variations with intermittent symptoms or with subacute symptoms.

Diagnosis

The classical features of vomiting, colicky pain, and constipation are usually easily recognized, though constipation may not become absolute for some time after the obstruction develops. General examination will also quickly show the degree of fluid and electrolyte loss as evidenced by skin laxity. sunken eyes, foetor, tachycardia and hypotension. Abdominal examination should be concentrated upon the patterns of visible peristalsis, left to right in the upper abdomen if gastric, ladder if small intestinal and flanks plus upper abdomen if colonic. Obstructive bowel sounds are typically high pitched and if absent indicate the presence of peritonitis. Early obstruction is relatively painless but if muscle guarding develops then strangulation, peritonitis and perforation must be considered. Apart from abdominal palpation for the presence of a mass, the hernial orifices must also be felt and the rectum examined digitally.

Plain abdominal X-rays will often show the obstructive lesion or site by gas contrast (barium contrast radiology should not be undertaken in the acute stage). The presence of one or two small fluid levels in an undistended bowel is of no significance.

Diagnosis of the pathological lesion is of comparatively minor importance and the section below gives a list of some of the commoner causes. If a diagnosis cannot be made pre-operatively little is lost if it is only made at laparotomy.

Causes of mechanical obstruction

Infants	Congenital anomalies, intussusception.
Young and middle-aged patients	Inflammatory lesions: appendicitis (also in the elderly).
Elderly patients	Neoplasm, diverticulitis, hernia, ischaemia, gallstones.
All ages	Swallowed foreign bodies, volvulus, adhesions.

Causes of functional obstruction

Steatorrhoea, debilitating medical illnesses (particularly with uraemia or hypotension), associated with peritonitis, diabetes mellitus, drugs (ganglion blocking agents), reflex effects of injury (e.g. spinal), hypokalaemia.

MANAGEMENT

The objects of treatment are to relieve the obstruction, reverse the complications and cure the cause.

Initial treatment should consist of intravenous infusion of fluids, intermittent gastric aspiration and relief of pain by drugs.

Assessment of fluid and electrolyte needs

Clinical. The duration of illness and the patient's account of the amounts of fluid lost, taken with clinical evidence of dehydration are the prime features.

Biochemical. Haemoglobin or packed cell volume, especially if known or expected to be normal previously, are valuable indices of dehydration. Extracellular dehydration also leads to reduced renal blood flow, urine flow, urea clearance and hence a rising blood urea. Urine examination for volume (especially in relation to time), specific gravity and salt content are also of great value. Diminished sodium or (as easily measured in the ward) chloride concentrations are good evidence of electrolyte depletion.

Fluid replacement

Deficits are commonly large, often in excess of 2 litres, and the aim should be to restore the circulating blood volume and at least part of extracellular fluid deficit before operation. Rapid infusion can be more easily controlled if central venous pressure is monitored through a superior vena caval catheter. The composition of secretions (Table 13) shows that all contain large amounts of electrolyte, especially sodium and chloride. In addition loss of gastric juice causes secondary impairment of renal function with abnormal loss of sodium ions. All gastro-intestinal losses should therefore be replaced with an isotonic sodium solution, commonly 0·9 per cent sodium chloride, which contains 140 mEq/litre of sodium. To this must be added potassium supplements as needed, low serum potassium concentrations are usually a good indication of deficit, though normal levels do not necessarily mean that there is no deficit. Disturbances of acid base balance rarely pose problems.

Table 13 Approximate electrolyte concentrations of gastrointestinal secretions (concentration, mEq/litre)

	H^+	Na^+	K^+	Cl^-	HCO_3^-
Gastric	60	60	9	100	0
Biliary	0	145	6	100	25
Pancreatic	0	110	5	50	30
Jejunal	0	140	6	138	6
Ileal	0	138	6	104	40
Colonic	0	139	13	103	50

Surgical treatment

Patients with acute obstruction, strangulation and closed loop obstruction need urgent operation. Daily assessment of those with other varieties of obstruction will show whether operation will be needed or not.

The prime reason for operation is to relieve the obstruction, but small intestinal causes of obstruction can usually be removed simultaneously. Colonic causes may demand staged procedures, classically in three phases with proximal colostomy, interval resection, and final operation for closure of the colostomy.

Two stage procedures have been advocated more recently and can considerably shorten hospital stay. They combine initial relieving colostomy with resection of the obstruction or else the second stage combines resection with closure of an initial relieving colostomy.

Chapter 7

LARGE BOWEL DISEASE

Constipation

Normal bowel habit varies from three bowel actions daily to two each week, and complaints of constipation and diarrhoea therefore need careful analysis.

Causes of decreased bowel frequency are shown in Table 14. Simple functional disease accounts for the problem in most cases, but the diagnosis must not be made without a full history, clinical, including rectal examination and appropriate investigations in adults and children alike.[84]

Management of constipation. In management a distinction should be drawn between slow intestinal transit—which can be

Table 14 Causes of constipation

Chronic constipation
1. Functional (a) with slow transit, idiopathic or low roughage content to diet, (b) with terminal reservoir syndrome.
2. Difficult or painful defaecation: pelvic muscular weakness; anal fissure
3. Pelvic tumours, e.g. fibroids
4. Intestinal obstructive lesions: carcinoma; aganglionosis, idiopathic megacolon
5. Iatrogenic: opiates, aluminium compounds etc
6. Toxic: lead poisoning
7. Metabolic and endocrine: myxoedema, hypercalcaemia, porphyria
8. Sense of incomplete evacuation: descending perineum syndrome

Acute constipation
1. Dehydration
2. Acute obstruction
3. Congenital lesions
4. Any of those causing chronic constipation

demonstrated using small radio-opaque polythene markers and the terminal reservoir syndrome in which the rectum appears to have a decreased sensitivity to distension.

In most cases with simple low transit and hard stools, a high residue diet supplemented by a bulk provider, such as methyl cellulose, and a liberal fluid intake will produce a regular formed soft stool. Rectal distension or insensitivity demands an effort to ensure that the patient allows sufficient time, preferably regularly each morning to defaecation and does not ignore the sensation of rectal distension. In the initial stages a contact laxative suppository such as bisacodyl and occasional doses of an osmotic purgative may be helpful.

Purgative drugs. There is a considerable array of laxative drugs available: and the main categories and some examples are shown below.

(a) Osmotic. Magnesium sulphate, lactulose.
(b) Lubricants. Liquid paraffin, dioctylsodium sulphosuccinate.
(c) Bulk producers. Methyl cellulose, Psyllium seeds.
(d) Stimulants. Bisacodyl, anthraquinones, e.g. Senna.
(e) Rectal preparations. Water and phosphate enemata, glycerine and bisacodyl suppositories.

The indications for continued use of any of these need to be examined carefully. Continued purgation can cause hypokalaemia and irritant purgatives such as senna and cascara can induce myenteric plexus damage[80] whilst oxyphenisatin, another irritant drug, has caused hepatic necrosis.

Laxative addiction. This unusual syndrome tends to occur in middle-aged women and should be considered when no obvious cause can be found for watery diarrhoea associated with hypokalaemia.[79] Small brown or black spots visible beneath the colonic mucosa (melanosis coli) should lead to suspicion of the use of anthraquinones. A search of the individual's belongings will usually reveal large amounts of laxatives, though patients can be very skilled in concealing evidence of their addiction.

Diarrhoea

A simple classification of causes of diarrhoea is shown in Table 15. Once correctable causes have been identified there remain a majority of patients with persistent symptoms of watery diarrhoea of unknown cause.

Table 15 Causes of diarrhoea

1. Functional: irritable bowel syndrome
2. Malabsorption syndromes (see Chapter 5)
3. Inflammatory disease: Crohn's disease, ulcerative colitis
4. Infections: bacterial, protozoal
5. Iatrogenic, e.g. magnesium compounds, laxative abuse, post vagotomy, antibiotic
6. Endocrine disorders: Thyrotoxicosis and medullary carcinoma[86], hypoparathyroidism, adrenogenital syndrome, Addison's disease, carcinoid syndrome, neural crest and islet cell tumours[85]
7. Metabolic disorders: uraemia, diabetes, congenital chloridorrhoea
8. Vascular disease
9. Allergy, e.g. milk protein
10. Spurious: faecal impaction, rectal tumours and inflammation
11. Postoperative: ileal resection

Standard drug therapy consists of the use of drugs which reduce intestinal motility, codein and diphenoxylate (Lomotil), preferably the former which is at least as effective as the latter, and cheaper. Kaolin is presumably effective because of its absorbent properties, and is especially valuable in the standard combination with morphine though somewhat bulky to handle.

DISORDERS OF WATER AND ELECTROLYTE HANDING

Cholerrheic enteropathy

Bile salts are normally mostly reabsorbed in the terminal ileum but if they pass into the colon are degraded to bile acids and are highly irritant to the bowel. They can then induce profuse watery diarrhoea by inhibiting salt and water absorption.[81]

Patients who have had ileocolonic resections for Crohn's disease, and ileocaecal tumours are particularly at risk.

Treatment. If codeine phosphate in the usual doses of 30–60 mg three time daily is unhelpful then the bile acid binding resin cholestyramine (Questran) is often effective.[82] Dosage requires careful individual titration as excessive amounts will cause steatorrhoea. It will also reduce absorption of other drugs especially thiazide diuretics, phenylbutazone and warfarin.

Congenital chloridorrhoea

This rare cause of watery diarrhoea is due to inability to secrete bicarbonate or to absorb chloride from the large bowel. Faecal chloride concentrations are consistently higher than sodium and potassium concentrations.

Diarrhoea and the sodium pump

The watery diarrhoea of cholera may be due to grossly overactive salt and electrolyte secretion but with normal absorption.[83] Since active sodium and in its turn water absorption in the small bowel are dependent upon glucose absorption, it was a logical step to determine whether oral glucose containing fluids would enhance absorption and mitigate the diarrhoea of cholera and perhaps other infective diarrhoeas. It now appears that choleraic diarrhoea can be treated by such oral therapy though whether other watery diarrhoeas can be so treated remains open to question.

FUNCTIONAL COLONIC DISORDERS

Irritable bowel syndrome

This is the commonest cause of lower bowel symptoms in Western populations, but the causes and mechanisms are poorly understood.

Aetiology and pathology. Important factors include the following.

(a) Postdysenteric irritability. Many patients can date symptom onset from a single sharp attack of (presumably) infective diarrhoea.

(b) Constitution. Many patients have histories of life-long bowel disturbance, and in some it is hard to discount the possibility of a relationship with personality problems.

(c) Directly related to other disorders e.g. with carbohydrate intolerance and postvagotomy.

(d) Secondary effects of other apparently unrelated disorders such as peptic ulcer, gallstones and gynaecological disease.

Mechanisms. Pressure studies using either miniature balloons passed through a sigmoidoscope or radiotelemetering devices occasionally show exaggerated responses in the colon following eating,[87] probably induced via a humoral pathway. The radiological counterpart is seen as an irregularly contractile but basically normal bowel which shows segmental hypermotility.

Clinical features and diagnosis. Symptoms vary from profuse watery diarrhoea with or without abdominal discomfort or colic through morning bowel frequency to, occasionally, a complete reversal with small constipated 'rabbit-like' stools. Despite these symptoms the patient's general health is good and physical examination and sigmoidoscopy are completely normal apart from the frequent demonstration of tenderness over the colon, and pain on rectal inflation.

The diagnosis is one of exclusion but the extent to which efforts are pressed must vary individually. There is, for instance, little to be gained from intensive investigation of young adults with mild symptoms.

Treatment. This is unsatisfactory and patients must be warned that symptoms will recur intermittently though they are especially likely to settle if there has been an initial attack of dysentery, or if a specific cause such as milk intolerance can be found and treated.[88] Bulk providers such as methyl cellulose and antidiarrhoeals such as codeine phosphate and diphenoxylate are helpful in relieving watery diarrhoea, whilst a high residue diet and again, methyl cellulose will help to relieve constipation. Anticholinergic drugs and the spasmolytic mebeverine will relieve pain.

Diverticular disease

Diverticula are frequently found on barium enema examination of patients over 40 years old in Western populations, the incidence rising increasingly with age, and the abnormalities being found especially often in the sigmoid colon.[89]

Aetiology and pathology. Colonic diverticula are herniations of mucosa through the muscular wall of the gut, and usually occur in rows related to the sites of muscular perforation by the arterial supply to the mucosa and submucosa at the antimesenteric taeniae coli. The factors causing herniation at these points are thought to include high intraluminal pressures generated by segmental muscular hyperactivity.

Pressure studies in the colon in patients with diverticulosis have (as in the irritable bowel syndrome) shown exaggerated responses to food and to injections of neostigmine and the muscle has been found at operation, or after death from other disease to be unduly thickened.

Increasing attention is being paid to the possibility that the diet of Western populations predisposes to such activity because of its low bulk content (Nigerian populations with a high bulk diet have been found by contrast to have little or no diverticulosis but a high incidence of sigmoid volvulus).[91]

Clinical features. There are four basic patterns, the first two being commonest.[90]

(a) Asymptomatic diverticulosis discovered incidentally.
(b) Symptomatic diverticulosis with complaints parallel to those in the irritable bowel syndrome.
(c) Diverticulitis. Acute inflammation probably initially due to faecolith impaction and followed by a varying degree of bacterial sepsis, including peridiverticulitis, pericolic abscess, ischiorectal abscess, fistulation, metastatic suppuration in the liver, perforation and general peritonitis.
(d) Sudden profuse painless rectal bleeding.

Diagnosis of diverticulosis is by barium enema with care to exclude neoplasm, by sigmoidoscopy and adequate films to examine the mucosal pattern of segments affected by the disease.

Diverticulitis usually gives rise to symptoms akin to left sided appendicitis with left sided pain, tenderness, fever and leucocytosis of sudden onset. Pericolic abscess should be suspected when there is a mass associated with obstruction. Right sided diverticulitis is uncommon and gives rise to confusion with, for instance, appendicitis and caecal neoplasm.

Medical treatment. Symptomless disease warrants no interference, but those with complaints similar to those of the irritable bowel syndrome need the same treatment.

Acute diverticulitis. Rest, with fluids only by mouth and treatment with a broad spectrum antibiotic (tetracycline or ampicillin) are usually adequate, though some dehydrated patients will need intravenous fluids.

Surgical treatment. Pericolic abscess needs drainage, and perforation requires closure as do fistulae. These procedures are combined appropriately with either relieving colostomy and later excision of the diseased area, or synchronous primary excision.

Symptomatic diverticulosis seldom requires operation but in

resistant cases, either resection of the affected area or (less conventionally) sigmoid myotomy of the thickened muscle are performed.

Congenital aganglionosis (Hirschsprung's disease)

Aetiology and pathology. The basic abnormality in this condition is a congenital lack of ganglion cells in the intramural plexus of the bowel wall causing loss of the normal peristaltic wave.

Clinical features. The disease is approximately ten times commoner in boys than in girls and usually manifests itself as severe constipation from birth onwards. The bowels may not be opened for weeks at a time and the general clinical picture is of intestinal obstruction with abdominal distension and vomiting and increased bowel sounds. When stools are passed they tend to be small and ribbon-like.

Barium enema will usually reveal a narrow rectum and a grossly dilated colon proximally, though occasionally the aganglionosis may extend into the small bowel. Rectal biopsy will usually provide a firm diagnosis, care being taken to include submucosal tissue.

Treatment. Symptoms vary considerably in severity and some neonates will require a relieving colostomy within days of birth. Other babies can be kept healthy for months by rectal washouts and occasional children with very mild disease may only present after several years.

Curative surgery has been based upon Swenson's procedure of rectosigmoidectomy with preservation of the anal sphincter, but the use of a number of variants attests to the occasional later problems of continued constipation, faecal soiling and interference with pelvic nerve function.

Other congenital anal abnormalities

These include complete absence of the anus, with the rectum ending in a blind pouch, imperforate anus with a simple obstructing membrane, and congenital anal stenosis. Absence of the anal canal is a rare condition requiring specialist surgery. Anal stenosis is more common and usually reponds to progressive dilatation.

Rectal inertia in childhood

Unlike congenital aganglionosis this usually presents several years after birth, is unassociated with distension, faecal soiling is common and rectal examination reveals a loaded rectum. It is frequently associated with psychiatric disturbance during the toilet training period.

Treatment involves disimpaction of rectal faecal masses followed by bowel re-education aided by simple enemata and contact laxatives such as bisacodyl, or senna.

Rectal prolapse

Partial or complete rectal mucosal prolapse occur as a result of repeated straining at stool, especially in elderly and debilitated people with defective pelvic and anal musculature.

Treatment is by replacement and, if necessary surgical removal of the excess mucosa and tightening of the anal sphincter.

Descending perineum syndrome

This consists of a sense of incomplete rectal evacuation with an urge to strain repeatedly. The anal sphincter is sited unduly low in relation to the pelvis or descends excessively on straining. The anterior rectal wall descends in particular and can be seen bulgin into a proctoscope as it is withdrawn. Explanation of the cause of symptoms, ensuring a soft normal bowel motion with mild laxatives, and if necessary injection treatment of the prolapsing mucosa are usually helpful.

Anal fissure

Sharp longitudinal narrow ulcers of the anal canal, anal fissures, are usually sited posteriorly, and tend to occur in the middle aged and elderly in association with constipation. The condition is often self-perpetuating because fear of painful defaecation leads to further constipation. Careful digital examination will usually reveal the lower end of the fissure (proctoscopy is very painful). Healing often follows with the use before defaecation of a local anaesthetic cream, and correction of any constipation. Chronic problems require anal dilatation and internal sphincterotomy, though care must be taken to avoid overenthusiastic surgery because of the hazard of faecal soiling due to the presence of an insensitive groove in the anal canal.

Internal piles

Aetiology and pathology. Rectal bleeding due to dilatation of the internal haemorrhoidal plexus of the superior haemorrhoidal veins is commonly caused by chronic constipation, pelvic swellings and occasionally develops in patients with chronic diarrhoea and in portal hypertension.

Clinical features. Rectal bleeding usually separate from and after a bowel motion are the classical features. But piles are so common that, particularly after the age of 40, a careful examination, including sigmoidoscopy, should be made to exclude other disease especially rectal tumours.

First degree (non-prolapsing) piles can usually be treated by perivenous injection of sclerosants. Second degree (occasionally prolapsing) or third degree (permanently prolapsed) piles usually require haemorrhoidectomy.

Painful prolapsed and thrombosed piles should be pressed gently back into the rectum under adequate analgesia or even general anaesthesia. The haemorrhoids should then be treated operatively once the inflammation has settled.

External piles

These are small peri-anal haematomata caused by subcutaneous vascular rupture. They are probably mainly caused by straining at stool in chronic constipation. Most resolve rapidly and uneventfully with conservative treatment.

Acquired megacolon due to Chagas' disease

Infection with South American trypanosomiasis may be followed by progressive loss of rectal and/or colonic ganglion cells, usually in adult life. The condition presents as a megacolon, and treatment is by excision of the diseased narrow segment.

Malrotation of the colon and incomplete descent of the caecum

These are usually found incidentally at barium enema examination. Volvulus is an occasional complication of malrotation.

Proctalgia fugax

Recurrent attacks of mild or severe rectal pain lasting up to a quarter of an hour, unassociated with organic disease are characteristic of this uncommon syndrome. Treatment is inadequate, attacks, which usually occur at night, may be prevented by taking an anticholinergic such as propantheline 30 mg before going to sleep. During the attack itself manual pressure on the anus or inflation of the rectum with a Higginson's syringe may abort the episode.

Solitary caecal ulcer

This rare condition tends to occur in an organ distended with faeces and the main feature is perforation.

Solitary rectal ulcer

Occasional patients complaining of rectal bleeding are found at sigmoidoscopy to have a single (and sometimes two or three) ulcers in the lower 10 cm of rectum. Histologically there is prominent fibroblastic invasion with cystic dilatation of crypts but normal mucosa elsewhere. The cause is unknown, it tends to be associated with constipation and in some patients is probably due to attempts at manual evacuation of the rectum.

Chapter 8

CROHN'S DISEASE

Pathology

The original concept of Crohn's disease as a non-specific inflammatory process affecting the terminal ileum has been widened and it is now accepted that any part of the gut may be affected.

Disease is predominantly ileal or colonic in site, extends submucosally with fissuring through muscle coats, granuloma formation and regional lymph node enlargement. Lesions may be discontinuous and multiple, diffuse or single.[92,93]

Epidemiology

Both sexes are affected equally and the incidence is greatest in young adults, the incidence rate being about 10 per cent of that of ulcerative colitis. The disease occurs in Jews and in families more often than can be accounted for by chance, but the causes are unknown. Though there are common histological features with sarcoidosis, and Kveim tests are often positive in Crohn's disease,[94] both diseases seem to occur separately. Experimental studies in mice suggest the presence of a transmissible, presumably infective factor, but no bacterial or other pathogen has ever been identified.[95] Evidence of hyporeactivity to immunological stimuli has also been obtained but the reasons for these changes are obscure.

Clinical features

Disease onset is insidious and patients ordinarily present with loose stools of a non-specific type, weight loss, lassitude, anaemia and lower abdominal pain. On examination there may be a palpable mass as well as tenderness and there may be features of associated disease or complications (see Table 16).

Table 16 Crohn's disease, complications and associated features

Complications

Commonly	1. Fistula	Usually peri-anal but it can be between small and large bowel, entero-enteral, vesical, vaginal or through the anterior abdominal wall
	2. Abscess	Associated with full thickness fissuring disease or peri-anal in site
	3. Stricture	Due to progressive inflammatory disease
	4. Gallstones	Due to ileal disease and bile salt deficiency
Less often	5. Carcinoma	Both small and large intestinal neoplasia have been described in association with Crohn's disease but the risk of neoplasm seems to be less than in ulcerative colitis
	6. Acute haemorrhage	
	7. Perforation	

Associated features

1. Skin disease	Erythema nodosum is a frequent concomitant of active Crohn's disease
2. Peri-anal lesions	Anal fissure or fistula is often a presenting feature; peri-anal lesions with bluish red mucosa undermined by relatively painless ulcers are a characteristic feature
3. Arthritis	Usually involving large joints and latex test negative
4. Ankylosing spondylitis	
5. Finger clubbing	
6. Liver disease	Non-specific fatty change or pericholangitis occasionally develops, and rarely cirrhosis
7. Uveitis and iritis	

The condition needs to be differentiated from ulcerative colitis, non-specific diarrhoeas, and from other causes of segmental inflammation such as tuberculosis and amoebiasis.

Barium meal or (preferably initially) barium enema will show areas of inflammatory change, segmental narrowing or stricture formation, which may be multiple with intervening normal mucosa. Occasionally there is diffuse involvement of the small bowel or colon. The radiological mucosal changes characteristically include deep fissuring of the bowel wall and fistulae occur in a minority of patients. The diagnosis can sometimes be confirmed by finding granulomata histologically in rectal biopsy specimens, occasionally even when the bowel looks normal to the naked eye.

Anaemia is commonly iron deficiency in type but megaloblastic change can occur with vitamin B_{12} deficiency (due to ileal disease or resection, or to the stagnant loop syndrome) and, more rarely, severe folate deficiency.

Hypoproteinaemia is due to exudative protein loss and gross oedema may be a feature of diffuse jejuno-ileal disease.

Diarrhoea may be steatorrhoeic, due to diffuse small intestinal disease or to bile salt deficiency with ileal disease or stagnant loop problems, and it can mimic that of ulcerative colitis.

Treatment

Adequate assessment of the value of medical treatments has been hampered by the difficulties of devising controlled trials in an uncommon disease with variable manifestations.

General supportive measures

Blood transfusion, and iron, folate and hydroxocobalamin may be needed to control anaemia, together with a high protein low fat diet in those with hypoproteinaemia and steatorrhoea. Codeine phosphate is helpful in controlling diarrhoea, and anticholinergic drugs in relieving pain.

Corticosteroid drugs. Though these are frequently used with apparently beneficial results, there is no objective evidence to support their use. Trial of prednisone 10 mg three or four times daily, tailing off slowly over several weeks, seems particularly worthwhile in those with diffuse jejuno-ileal disease, with slow progressive deterioration, or who have relapsed after operation. They should be avoided in patients with strictures, abscesses or (usually) fistulae.

Sulphasalazine. Benefit is often claimed from its use but has no support. Sulphasalazine can be justified on the analogy of its usefulness in colitis and because it, unlike steroids, seldom has serious side effects in long term use.

Antibiotics. These have a clear place in treating infective complications and the stagnant loop syndrome but it is doubtful if they have any other value.

Immunosuppressives. Favourable responses to treatment with azathioprin have been recorded in several uncontrolled investigations and in one controlled trial.[96] However, this result is counterbalanced by another negative controlled comparison.[97] Further evidence is required before widespread use can be recommended.

Surgery and prognosis

The prime indications for operation are complications of stricture, abscess and fistula. Most patients come to operation either with these problems or because it is hoped that resection will relieve symptoms due to an isolated disease segment. Unfortunately recurrence rates are high after apparently successful operations and since disease does tend to become inactive as time passes a reasonably conservative approach seems justified.

Operations. Resection and anastomosis seems preferable to bypass in that problems due to retained active disease and stagnant loop syndromes are avoided.[98-100] Recurrence rates are still high, however (Table 17), and death either from complications or due to progressive loss of bowel is not uncommon.

Table 17 Relapse rate after resection of Crohn's disease[99]

	No. studied	Cumulative relapse rate (%)
Within 1 year	168	15·5
Within 5 years	79	22·5
Within 9 years	69	35·3

COLONIC CROHN'S DISEASE

The essential distinction between Crohn's disease of the colon and ulcerative colitis is pathological and the main contrasting features are shown in Table 18.

Table 18 Comparative features of Crohn's disease and ulcerative colitis

	Crohn's disease	Ulcerative colitis
Disease features	Segmental (usually)	Diffuse continuous
Rectal involvement	Often absent	Usually present
Inflammation	Full thickness	Mucosal
Crypt abscesses	Less frequent	Common
Granulomata	Present	Absent
Peri-anal lesions	Frequent	Infrequent
Small intestinal disease	Often present	Absent

Medical treatment. It is accepted, though without any objective evidence in support, that sulphasalazine and corticosteroids are beneficial in colonic Crohn's disease as well as ulcerative colitis. Immunosuppressive agents may possibly be useful but still form an experimental treatment.

Surgical treatment. Limited resections or ileorectal anastomosis are often possible in colonic Crohn's disease but recurrence rates are in general very high and are equally so in patients with diffuse colonic Crohn's disease requiring ileostomy.

Chapter 9

ULCERATIVE COLITIS AND ISCHAEMIC COLITIS

ULCERATIVE COLITIS

Non-specific inflammatory disease of the large bowel forms a distinct clinical entity which can be recognized separately from other varieties of colonic inflammatory disease such as diverticulitis and Crohn's disease (Table 18).

Pathology

The characteristic features are of diffuse inflammatory change. largely, if not totally confined to the mucosa, usually maximal in the rectum and spreading proximally and to a variable degree towards the ileocaecal valve but no more than 1–2 cm beyond it. Histological examination shows a variable degree of mucosal destruction and infiltration with polymorphs, eosinophils and, particularly in the chronic stages, with plasma cells and lymphocytes. Epithelial crypts frequently become full of inflammatory cells forming crypt abscesses. During healing the mucosa may form irregular projections (pseudo-polyps) as the epithelial surface regenerates over exuberant granulation tissue and crypts may become apparently branched rather than remaining single parallel structures. In severe acute disease inflammatory change may involve the muscle and the wall may perforate or in the long term be converted into an inert fibrous epithelial lined tube.

Epidemiology and causation

The disease can present at any age, but usually in early adult life, and is about twice as common in women as men and in Jews compared with non-Jews. It also tends to appear in family aggregates. Ulcerative colitis incidence rates are approximately ten times those of Crohn's disease in Western communities. It is rarely diagnosed in the tropics but this may be due to confusion with endemic infective dysenteries rather than truly low incidence rates.

The cause of ulcerative colitis is unknown but the mucosal infiltration with plasma cells and lymphocytes, clinical response to steroid treatment and the detection of circulating anticolon antibodies all suggest an immune basis.[101] Cross reaction between these antibodies and serological sub-types of *E. coli* further suggest that an inappropriate antibacterial response may be implicated. There is no good evidence to support a simple infective cause and attempts to establish a primary psychosomatic basis have been unconvincing.

Clinical features[102]

Lower bowel symptoms of frequent loose bowel motions containing blood and mucus are by far the most prominent characteristics. The onset may be slow and insidious or dramatically severe, may be associated with moderately severe or negligible abdominal pain, and with much or little constitutional disturbance with anaemia, weight loss and fever.

Physical examination in mild cases shows no abnormality, except perhaps tenderness over the colon, but sigmoidoscopy will reveal the characteristic changes of diffuse inflammation of varying degree. If mild there may be little more than loss of the normal appearance of a ramifying vascular submucosal pattern and replacement by diffuse granularity with easy contact bleeding. If severe there will be obvious free blood and mucopus in the lumen. Mucosal biopsy should in general be undertaken for it will help in distinguishing doubtful visual changes from those, for instance, due to simple acute diarrhoea, and will give permanent documentary support to the visual report. The extent of disease can often be determined sigmoidoscopically, and in those with disease proximal to the rectosigmoid barium enema will confirm the presence and extent of diffuse proximal inflammatory change. Early abnormalities consist of loss of the normal sharp mucosal outline and later include loss of haustral pattern, irregular mucosal outline due to pseudo-polyposis and finally conversion to a smooth atonic fibrous tube.

In severe disease there may be gross anaemia of iron deficiency type, wasting, hypoproteinaemia, dehydration and electrolyte disturbance with salt and potassium deficiencies. Other associated clinical features are shown in Table 19. Of these skin, liver, eye and joint disease usually settle simultaneously as the colonic disease either becomes inactive or is treated surgically, but any of them may present several months or years before the apparent onset of colitis.

Table 19 Associated features and complications of ulcerative colitis

Associated features
1. Skin disease	Erythema nodosum and pyoderma gangrenosum
2. Arthritis	Involving large joints (few simultaneously) and latex negative
3. Ankylosing spondylitis and sacro-iliitis	
4. Finger clubbing	
5. Liver disease	Fatty change, pericholangitis, chronic active hepatitis, abscess, and (rarely) carcinoma of the bile duct
6. Iritis and uveitis	

Complications
1. Toxic megacolon, perforation, severe acute bleeding
2. Carcinoma of colon
3. Benign stricture
4. Ischiorectal abscess

Treatment

Management varies greatly according to the severity and type of disease. Patients with localized proctitis may need nothing more than occasional courses of outpatient treatment with steroid suppositories whilst those with severe generalized disease are at risk of the complications listed in Table 19 particularly the first, toxic megacolon.[103]

Mild attacks

Anti-inflammatory drugs (Table 20).

Sulphasalazine. There is good controlled trial evidence that this is beneficial in suppressing mild active disease. In doses of

1 g three or four times daily dose related side effects of nausea, vomiting and anorexia are seldom prominent though allergic skin rashes can cause abandonment of treatment.

Table 20 Outpatient treatment of mildly to moderately severe ulcerative colitis (to help in comparability all results refer to trials conducted at one centre)

Active disease
Oral Prednisone three different doses for 3 weeks[104]

	No. studied	Percentage remission
20 mg daily	20	25
40 mg daily	20	55
60 mg daily	20	65

Retention enemata for 4 weeks[105]

	No. studied	Percentage remission
Prednisone 21 phosphate (20 mg nightly)	34	50
Betamethasone valerate (5 mg nightly)	36	50

Prophylaxis after remission
Sulphasalazine (2 g daily) or placebo for 12 months[106]

	No. studied	Percentage relapsing
Sulphasalazine	30	20
Placebo	32	75

Prednisone 15 mg daily or placebo for 6 months[107]

| Prednisone | 30 | 60 |
| Placebo | 29 | 59 |

Local steroids. Prednisolone 21 phosphate (Predsol) suppositories (10 mg) or enemata (20 mg in a 100 ml disposable enema bag) are effective treatments, given on going to bed to be retained until the morning if possible, for respectively lower rectal and rectosigmoid inflammatory disease. Predsol retention enemata are absorbed systemically to some extent and will suppress endogenous steroid output. Betamethasone retention enemata have the (theoretical) advantage of preventing such suppression, though it is doubtful if this is clinically significant.

Oral steroids. Prednisone in oral doses of 20 to 40 mg daily will induce remission in 2–4 weeks in most patients and is to be preferred for outpatient treatment of moderately severe attacks in patients who have more extensive disease, or who cannot manage to retain enemata.

Supportive measures. A high protein diet, codeine phosphate for diarrhoea and anticholinergic drugs for pain are standard ancillary measures. Iron deficiency anaemia is probably better treated with a slow release iron preparation such as Slow Fe (Ciba) as many colitics get bowel upset with standard iron preparations.

Severe attacks

Patients with severe diarrhoea and constitutional disturbance should be treated in hospital. Oral sulphasalazine has little or no place in such circumstances and rectal steroids are not always well enough retained to be useful as the sole treatment.

Systemic steroid treatment should be given as prednisone 10–15 mg four times daily by mouth or as ACTH gel or long acting synthetic corticotrophin 40–60 units twice daily by injection. ACTH has given higher remission rates than corticosteroids in the past in very severe disease but it is uncertain whether this reflects dosage effects or perhaps poor absorption of oral steroids. ACTH is therefore generally recommended for bad attacks. Intravenous fluid and electrolyte replacement may be required and patients should be transfused if haemoglobin concentrations fall below 10 grams per cent.

Complications of acute disease

Toxic megacolon. Patients with extensive acute disease occasionally develop progressive dilatation of part (usually the transverse segment) of the colon. This condition, toxic megacolon, if unrecognized will progress to perforation and mortality rates then rise to 50 per cent or more. Those individuals with severe attacks who have slight abdominal distension or percussable gas in the bowel should have plain radiographs taken. The large (6 cm or more in transverse diameter) gas filled shadow of a toxic megacolon is instantly recognizable. When this complication occurs or is thought likely all oral intake except water or fruit juices should be stopped, and intravenous therapy given with adequate blood, fluid and electrolyte content. In addition patients should receive ACTH 40–60 u twice daily and a broad spectrum antibiotic such as tetracycline or ampicillin parenterally in the hope of minimizing any septicaemia. At this stage surgical co-operation, but not necessarily intervention, should be sought and the patient closely watched, with daily plain radiographs for 2–3 days. Less than half of all patients will settle in this time and if not then emergency ileostomy and panproctocolectomy should be undertaken. A policy of early surgical intervention has considerably lowered the death rate compared with prolonged medical treatment (Table 21).

Table 21 Result of treatment including an early surgical policy in eighty patients with severe acute ulcerative colitis[109]

Medical treatment and remission	38
Early surgery	43
Total deaths	1

Prevention of relapse (Table 20).

Corticosteroids. Neither cortisone, 50 mg daily nor prednisone 15 mg daily have been shown to prevent relapse, and steroid treatment should always be tailed off once an acute attack has settled.

Sulphasalazine. There is good controlled trial evidence that this drug will prevent relapse when given in a dose of 0·5 g four times daily.

Immunosuppressive drugs. There is as yet no conclusive evidence that these are effective in preventing relapse.

Milk free diet. An unusually high proportion of colitic patients have circulating antibodies to milk protein and a milk free diet seems to help a minority of patients. This may be through relieving minor degrees of lactose intolerance rather than any immunological effect.

Prognosis

Less than 10 per cent of patients present with severe or fulminating disease and mortality in both the short and long term is greatest in this group. Most patients, even those with mild disease have recurrent attacks, 80 per cent having second episodes within a year of their first attack. However, a few patients remain symptom free for many years after a single attack and those with minor disease, commonly sigmoidoscopically characteristic but radiologically normal, have a good long term prognosis. Disease usually is then non-progressive and mortality experience little if at all different from that of the rest of the population.[108]

Surgery

No operation less than colectomy is worthwhile; the generally accepted procedure is panproctocolectomy with ileostomy but ileorectal anastomosis has its advocates despite the problems of local recurrence and occasionally carcinoma.

Indications for operation

Acute attacks: (a) failed medical treatment, but without undue delay;[109] (b) toxic megacolon and perforation.

Chronic disease: (a) Continuous symptoms or recurrent attacks preventing normal life activity; (b) Proven, suspected, or likely complications of carcinoma; (c) Management of progressive disabling extrabowel complications—especially arthritis.

Whenever possible patients having ileostomies performed should have the opportunity to discuss the procedure with a member of the Ileostomy Association. The mortality from elective surgery in good hands is about 2 per cent but this can rise over tenfold if operation is precipitated by severe acute disease. Postoperative complications are probably more common in patients who have had much corticosteroid therapy (which must be continued over operation and tailed off gradually thereafter).

Risk of carcinoma

Ulcerative colitis of ten years duration and when extensive (spreading proximal to the splenic flexure) has a high risk of malignant change (Table 22). A case can therefore be made out for elective total colectomy in those at such risk. Atypical and unstable mucosal changes may be helpful in defining which patients are especially at risk, but in general any relapse in patients with diffuse longstanding disease should raise the possibility of neoplastic change.

Table 22 Risk of cancer in ulcerative colitis

(a) *Influence of disease extent*[108]

Bowel involvement by colitis	No. of cases of colitis	Percentage developing cancer*
Total	236	7·2
Partial	388	1·3

(b) *Influence of disease duration*[109]

Duration of symptoms (years)	No. of cases of colitis	Percentage annual risk of cancer**
1–9	151	0·4
10–19	33	2·0
20 or more	26	5·8

(Continuous or initially severe symptoms and paediatric onset are not predisposing factors.)

*At any time in disease course
**With extensive bowel disease only

Prognosis

Despite steroid treatment there is still a considerable mortality rate with severe or progressive colitis. Once operation has been performed, the life expectancy and general health of ileostomists are similar to those of the rest of the community[110] except in two respects.[111] There is an increased risk of renal stones (due to their more delicate fluid balance) and there is a risk of impotence due to pelvic nerve injury in men at rectal excision. For this reason some surgeons tend to defer rectal excision in young men.

ISCHAEMIC COLITIS

Aetiology and pathology

This uncommon cause of colon disease, probably less frequent than colonic Crohn's disease, presents in patients over 50 years old, and is due to thrombosis or embolism of the mesenteric vessels.[112] It is usually segmental and characteristically affects the splenic flexure where the arterial supply is particularly precarious.[113,114]

Clinical features and treatment

The sudden onset of abdominal pain with rectal bleeding and diarrhoea should give rise to suspicion of the condition. If severe, gangrene of the bowel will supervene. Less dramatic cases will settle gradually and the diagnosis can usually be made early in the disease by barium enema when there is characteristically a regular segmental thumb printing abnormality due to oedematous swelling.

Sigmoidoscopy will be normal unless (uncommonly) rectal ischaemia has caused inflammatory change. With healing there is muscular replacement by fibrous tissue and a stricture may form.

Chapter 10

PERITONEAL DISORDERS

PERITONITIS

Pathology. It usually occurs secondary to some obvious abnormality, irritation or infection, but occasionally may arise as an apparently isolated condition, for instance due to pneumococcal infection. Causes of peritonitis include the following:
(a) Gut perforation, secondary to peptic ulcer, or to perforation of an inflamed organ as in appendicitis, diverticulitis, cholecystitis and ulcerative colitis.
(b) Spread from the female genital tract, as in salpingitis.
(c) Circulatory spread of infection occurring elsewhere in the body or apparent primary disease.
(d) Secondary to penetrating wounds, either through simple trauma, or occasionally postoperatively or following needle biopsy or percutaneous cholangiography in jaundice.

Due to natural anatomical boundaries peritonitis may localize in four main areas, (a) and (b) laterally on either side of the boundary formed by the spine, its related structures and small intestinal mesentery, (c) within the pelvis and (d) above the transverse colon.

Clinical features. Acute perforation of a hollow viscus such as a peptic ulcer is almost always followed by the sudden onset of severe pain, associated with vomiting, prostration, marked abdominal tenderness, rigidity and loss of bowel sounds. Sometimes infection, for instance in the pelvis or in appendicitis is localized by adhesions and signs of generalized peritonitis do not occur. Instead a tender mass develops usually with paralytic ileus and a swinging fever. In most cases of acute peritonitis there is constipation, but pelvic infections may be associated initially with diarrhoea.

Peritonitis associated with tuberculous infection is seldom

painful, and is often confused with a malignant ascites. Bacterial infection of cirrhotic ascites is also relatively painless, the diagnosis being suspected because of an unexplained fever, and in ulcerative colitis there is frequently relief of pain when a toxic megacolon perforates.

Management. Focal conditions causing peritonitis demand surgical treatment, together with antibiotic therapy and adequate intravenous fluid and electrolyte replacement. Primary peritonitis, infected ascites and tuberculous peritonitis need appropriate antibiotic treatment without operation. Tuberculous infection is often hard to diagnose with complete certainty for ascitic fluid is often sterile on culture, and tuberculin skin tests may sometimes be negative and chest X-ray normal. Peritoneal biopsy may reveal tubercles but if the diagnosis is suspected but unproven then a trial of triple chemotherapy with streptomycin, PAS and isoniazid is clearly justified.

SUBPHRENIC ABSCESS

This may complicate any infection within the right paracolic gutter. It is a well recognized complication of perforated peptic ulcer and upper abdominal surgery but may also occur secondary to supradiaphragmatic infection and to rupture of a liver abscess.

Clinical features: these include swinging fever, pain in the right upper abdomen, or referred to the right shoulder, hiccup, and polymorphonuclear leucocytosis. Radiology will show a raised right diaphragm with or without a small pleural effusion and sometimes a fluid level in the abscess.

Management. Extraperitoneal surgical drainage (to prevent general peritoneal spread) is essential, usually together with antibiotic treatment.

LYMPHADENITIS

(a) Tuberculous. This is usually diagnosed retrospectively because calcified abdominal glands are noted radiologically. No treatment is then required.

(b) Non-specific varieties. Right sided abdominal pain, commonly mimicking symptoms of acute appendicitis, is the usual feature. Operation (undertaken to ensure that appendicitis is not present) reveals enlarged mesenteric lymph nodes only. In some

individuals the condition seems to be due to infection with *Yersinia enterocolitica*:[77] no treatment is required as remission is usually quick and uneventful.

PERITONEAL TUMOURS

Secondary malignant deposits are by far the commonest variety and multiple seedling deposits (the usual type) cause ascites. The diagnosis may be obvious (for instance in known gastric cancer) or it may only be made by laparotomy. Malignant cells are often hard to detect with confidence in diagnostic aspirates, but a high protein concentration should lead to suspicion of tuberculosis or malignancy.

Rapid reaccumulation of fluid can sometimes be retarded by intraperitoneal chemotherapy, for instance with radioactive gold.

PSEUDOMYXOMA PERITONEI

Ruptured ovarian cystadenoma or appendix mucocoele may cause seeding of the peritoneum with cells which form large gelatinous deposits and cause ascites. General health is well preserved despite the ascites, and the other hallmark is difficulty in aspirating the mucilaginous material. When treatment by aspiration is impractical, operative clearance of as much material as possible and radioactive gold, or cytotoxic drug treatment intraperitoneally are required.

OMENTAL TORSION

This rarely occurs as a primary disorder, and usually follows adhesion of the omentum to the parietal peritoneum. The patient presents with abdominal pain as a typical acute abdominal emergency. It is sometimes associated with a high serum amylase—without pancreatitis.

Treatment is by resection of the twisted omentum.

MESENTERIC CYSTS

Cysts usually occur in childhood or early adult life and cause symptoms if they become very large or twist on their pedicles. Treatment is by operative removal.

FAMILIAL MEDITERRANEAN FEVER
(PERIODIC DISEASE)

The disease is characterized by recurrent fever associated with abdominal pain, which may simulate that of peritonitis but can last for several weeks and is often associated with arthralgia, pleuritic pain and urticaria. It usually occurs in patients of Mediterranean or Armenian stock, commonly Jews and the cause is unknown.

Treatment. No specific measures are available and once the diagnosis is made (by exclusion of other specific causes of pain) intermittent corticosteroid therapy may be needed. The prognosis is good except when complications of amyloidosis or lymphoma develop—as they commonly do in the East, but curiously seldom elsewhere.

Chapter II

GASTROINTESTINAL CANCER AND POLYPOSIS

OESOPHAGEAL CANCER

Aetiology and epidemiology

This tumour varies by up to fiftyfold in frequency throughout the world and is virtually always commoner in men than women, though the sex ratio fluctuates considerably (see Table 23). Patterns of high and low incidence vary erratically and grossly over short distances geographically—especially in Africa—and almost certainly reflect the dominant importance of

Table 23 *Age standardized incidence rates per 100,000 population per year and male to female ratios in gastric and oesophageal cancer*[115]

	Oesophagus			Stomach		
	Men	Women	Ratio	Men	Women	Ratio
Puerto Rico	18·0	7·7	2·3:1	29·0	13·6	2·2:1
Japan	13·4	6·3	2·1:1	95·5	47·7	2·0:1
Iceland	8·5	6·2	1·4:1	70·0	30·1	2·3:1
Finland	7·1	5·8	1·2:1	53·2	29·5	1·8:1
England and Wales (four regions)	4·5	2·4	1·9:1	24·8	12·4	2·0:1
U.S.A. (New York state)	4·2	1·0	4·2:1	13·7	6·6	2·1:1

environmental factors on tumour incidence. Smoking and alcohol consumption are both associated with liability to oesophageal cancer but no specific causal factor has yet been confidently identified.[116]

Predisposing diseases

(a) Achalasia of the cardia, especially if inadequately treated, predisposes to the late development of oesophageal tumours presumably due to chronic irritation.
(b) Iron deficiency anaemia can lead to hypopharyngeal tumours as well as oesophageal webs.
(c) Tylosis, a rare condition of dyskeratosis of the soles of the feet and palms of the hands is very occasionally associated with liability to oesophageal neoplasia, and is then inherited as a Mendelian dominant. (Hiatus hernia and oesophagitis are not predisposing factors.)

Clinical features

The classical symptoms are of dysphagia which is of short duration, remorselessly progressive, initially for solid foods but soon including liquids. This has to be distinguished from the dysphagia of oesophageal stricture (Chapter 1) and achalasia.

Diagnosis

Barium swallow will usually reveal the characteristic features of irregular luminal narrowing often of a 'rats-tail' appearance. Oesophagoscopic confirmation is easily obtained.

Pathology

Most tumours involve the lower third of the gullet and are squamous. Adenocarcinomata of the lower end of the oesophagus should be considered as primary gastric tumours, though occasional adenocarcinomata arise in oesophageal mucous glands.

Treatment

Oesophageal tumours infiltrate early and widely, and apparently complete operative removal is depressingly infrequent (Table 24). Operation has a high early mortality and late death from metastases is common. Radiotherapy may well offer equally good (but still poor overall) curative results and palliation by intubation of the malignant stricture is often the best that can be done.

Table 24 Five-year survival rates in patients with gastrointestinal cancer diagnosed in 1962–63, Sheffield Regional Hospital Board Area[118]

	No. diagnosed	Percentage survival overall	No. treatable	Percentage survival
Oesophagus	325	3	185	6
Stomach	1924	6	784	12
Colon	1516	26	1072	36
Rectum	1263	28	961	35

GASTRIC CANCER

Aetiology and epidemiology

Cancer of the stomach varies in frequency by a factor of approximately tenfold throughout the world but in all areas it is approximately twice as common in men as in women (Table 23) and in all areas it increases steadily in incidence with advancing age. No specific causal dietary or other factor has been identified, but comparisons of world incidence patterns and changes in incidence in migrants from one country to another suggest that environmental influences are of paramount importance. There is also a minor genetic factor, the disease, like pernicious anaemia being slightly more common in individuals of blood group A then in those of the remaining ABO blood groups.

Predisposing diseases

Gastric cancer is roughly four times commoner in those with pernicious anaemia than in the general population, and it may also have a slightly increased frequency in any person with chronic atrophic gastritis[117] or after partial gastrectomy. Multiple gastric adenomatous polyps are also probably premalignant. Gastric ulcer does not predispose to cancer and any apparent link is on the basis of misdiagnosis, or perhaps a common gastric soil.

Pathology

Adenocarcinomata of the stomach metastasize early and irregularly by the lymphatic system and through the blood stream. Submucosal infiltration (linitis plastica) also occasionally occurs. Other varieties of malignant tumour—lymphomata and sarcomata—are rare, making up 5 per cent or less of the total tumour incidence.

Clinical features

Apart from pain of ulcer type, loss of appetite and weight loss are important warning symptoms, acute haemorrhage or chronic anaemia are also presenting features. Antral tumours often cause pyloric obstruction whilst fundal growths can cause dysphagia. A palpable mass is only felt in a minority of patients, though presentation with liver metastases and with metastatic glands, particularly in the left supraclavicular triangle of the neck (Virchow's node) is well recognized.

Diagnosis

Barium meal examination will reveal tumours as filling defects or ulcers, and will also detect submucosal infiltrating tumours by the undue rigidity they give to the stomach. Gastroscopy especially when combined with direct vision biopsy is valuable in confirming the diagnosis and in distinguishing benign from malignant ulcers. Exfoliative cytology is of limited value even to the experienced and gastric function tests are almost useless. Hypochlorhydria with cancer cannot be distinguished from hypochlorhydria with increasing age, though complete achlorhydria with a gastric ulcer is virtually diagnostic of cancer in the few patients where this combination can be found.

Treatment

Surgical excision offers the only hope of cure because radiotherapy and chemotherapy are ineffective (as in all adenocarcinomata of the gut) except in the few patients with primary gastric lymphomata which are too extensive for excision. However, the pattern of early and irregular metastasis is associated with poor long or even short term surgical results (Table 24). The best prognosis is found in the few who have growths limited to the mucosa, often misdiagnosed operatively as simple ulcers and in those with pronounced lymphocytic invasion of the tumour.

SMALL INTESTINAL TUMOURS

Adenocarcinomata

These form only 1 per cent of gastrointestinal tumours, and present with obstruction, weight loss and obscure anaemia. Their cause is unknown. Isolated cases have been described with pre-existing Crohn's disease and this may represent a true association. Treatment is by operation.

Lymphomata

Single multiple or diffusely spreading lymphomata can occur in isolation and are also recognized complications of coeliac disease. They usually present with symptoms of anaemia and diarrhoea (particularly as 'resistant' coeliac syndrome). One rare variety is associated with a dysgammaglobulinaemia (alpha chain disease). Though in theory responsive to chemo- and radiotherapy the prognosis is, in practice, very poor.

Carcinoid tumours

Clinical features

These are frequently found in the appendix, but they can also occur widely elsewhere in the gastrointestinal tract, and in the lung and ovary.

Carcinoid tumours are very slow growing, and metastasize late. Most are found incidentally at operation for other reasons but occasionally they can cause intestinal obstruction.

Malignant carcinoid syndrome. Small intestinal (midgut) carcinoid tumours but curiously not large intestinal or appendicular (hindgut) tumours can secrete a variety of substances including 5-hydroxytryptamine, kallikrein and bradykinin. Such tumours are readily recognized by the rusty red granules seen on diazo staining of formalin fixed tissues. When metastases are present in the liver serotonin and other active substances are released into the systemic circulation and give rise to the striking clinical features of episodic flushing, telangiectasia, watery diarrhoea, bronchospasm and right sided cardiac valve abnormalities.

Diagnosis

Malignant intestinal carcinoid syndrome is invariably associated with hepatomegaly due to the metastases. 5-Hydroxyindoleacetic acid a metabolite of 5-hydroxytryptamine can also be detected in the urine. Precipitation of flushing by microgram injections of adrenalin is a useful manoeuvre in doubtful cases.

Treatment

Surgical resection is impossible because of the extensive metastases though removal of an isolated large secondary deposit sometimes helps palliate symptoms. Useful palliation of symptoms may also be obtained with methysergide 2 mg three times daily, or *p*-chlorophenylalanine[119,120] which block activity of the tumour products. They are usually more effective in suppressing diarrhoea than flushing.

Prognosis

Patients may survive many years despite extensive metastases. Regional perfusion of the liver with cytotoxic drugs may therefore be worthwhile in palliating symptoms when simple blocking drug treatment fails.

COLONIC AND RECTAL CANCER

Aetiology and epidemiology

Colonic cancer is slightly more common in women than men, whereas rectal cancer is more common in men than women. Both tend to increase in frequency with age and to vary in geographical frequency in inverse ratio with cancer of the stomach. The causes of large intestinal cancer are completely unknown but environmental and presumably dietary factors are of paramount importance.

Predisposing diseases

Ulcerative colitis (when extensive, and prolonged in duration) and familial polyposis coli are well proven premalignant conditions but account for only a very small proportion of all cases recorded.

Clinical features

Both varieties of large intestinal cancer commonly present as disorder of bowel habit with or without abdominal pain or intestinal obstruction. In addition tumours in the colon occasionally intussuscept and carcinoma of the caecum can present as iron deficiency anaemia of apparently obscure cause. Carcinoma of the rectum commonly gives rise to rectal bleeding with urgency and much mucus production.

Diagnosis

Seventy-five per cent of all large bowel carcinomata are sited in the rectum and rectosigmoid so that sigmoidoscopic examination is essential whenever the diagnosis is suspected. Barium enema examination will distinguish tumours above the rectosigmoid but there are inevitably difficulties in distinguishing tumours from filling defects due to retained faeces in an ill prepared bowel and from spastic areas associated with diverticular disease. Where the diagnosis is doubtful double contrast barium enema studies and colonoscopy with a flexible end-viewing fiberscope help in assessing high (suprarectal) lesions. A tumour associated antigenic glycoprotein (carcino-embryonic antigen), has been found especially often in the serum of colonic cancer patients and may ultimately form the basis of an immunological diagnostic test.[121,122] It can also be found (in small amounts) in normal serum, in patients with other cancers, and in general in cancer the amount increases with tumour extent.

Treatment

Wherever possible tumours should be excised. Abdomino-perineal resection with left iliac fossa colostomy is necessary for tumours sited within 10 cm of the anal margin. Continuity of the bowel can usually be restored with higher lesions, though a staged procedure, with preliminary decompressing colostomy may be needed when tumours have presented with intestinal obstruction.

Prognosis

Unlike other varieties of gastrointestinal cancer, the prognosis of cancer of the colon and rectum is related strongly and simply to the amount of spread present at operation (Table 25).

Table 25 Prognosis of rectal cancer (resectable cases)[123]

	No. of patients	Percentage 5-year survival
Limited to rectal mucosa	308	97·7
Local spread through the muscle wall only	692	77·6
Lymph node invasion	1037	32·0

OTHER, UNCOMMON, TUMOURS OF THE LARGE BOWEL

Squamous cell carcinoma of the anal verge. This must be differentiated from perianal Crohn's disease (which is a characteristic blue undermined ulcerating lesion), tuberculosis, primary chancre and simple anal fissure. Treatment is surgical with or without local radiotherapy.

Sarcoma, carcinoid and lymphoma. All these can present as primary large intestinal tumours: treatment is identical with that for varieties detected elsewhere.

HEPATIC CARCINOMA

Malignant tumours

Secondary carcinomata are many times commoner than primary hepatomata in Western countries, but in parts of Africa and elsewhere primary tumours may be commoner than all other varieties of malignancy combined.

Primary hepatoma

Aetiology and pathology

Most develop secondary to cirrhosis in Europeans but in Africans there is usually no pre-existing disease. It is known, however, that a variety of carcinogens will induce liver cancer, and one possible cause in man is aflatoxin, a toxic product of aspergilli which cause mould diseases of peanuts and other carbohydrate foods.

Pathologically most are tumours of parenchymal origin but some are derived from cholangiolar tissue. Spread occurs by direct infiltration, and by the bloodstream and lymphatic systems.

Clinical features

These include upper abdominal pain with tender hepatomegaly, and ascites with blood stained fluid. Diagnosis may be difficult, but scintiscanning may show a filling defect in the liver and malignant cells may be found in ascitic fluid. Recently it has been found that alpha foetoprotein, a globulin which usually disappears from the circulation at birth, is detectable serologically in primary liver cancer. The frequency varies from under 50 per cent of cases in the United Kingdom and U.S.A. to 75 per cent or more in tropical areas, presumably reflecting aetiological differences. The presence of foetoprotein is a strong indication of liver cancer, for no other tumour has yet been shown to be associated with similar abnormalities, except testicular teratoblastoma in 10 per cent of cases,[124] (and also, curiously, pyridoxine deficiency[125]).

Treatment

Hepatic lobectomy is occasionally possible, hepatic arteriography being needed as well as scintiscanning to define the lesion. Regional perfusion with cytotoxic agents can occasionally give useful palliation, but liver transplantation is an experimental procedure. In most cases simple palliation is the wisest (and kindest) measure.

Secondary carcinomata

These usually arise from gut, breast, bronchus and reproductive organs. Scintiscanning, with later liver biopsy if necessary, are the best diagnostic procedures but serum alkaline phosphatase and 5′ nucleotidase estimations are reasonable screening measures.

Treatment by resection is rarely possible and cytotoxic agents are seldom helpful, it is better to help the patient to die peacefully.

Rarer tumours causing specific problems are metastasizing carcinoids and insulinomata.

CARCINOMA OF THE PANCREAS

Aetiology and pathology

The causes of this common intra-abdominal tumour (forming 9 per cent of all gastrointestinal malignancies in the United Kingdom and the U.S.A.) are unknown.

Adenocarcinomata. These are by far the most frequent variety. Most are found in the head of the pancreas and one third in the body and tail. Local invasion of the pancreas causes biliary and pancreatic duct obstruction by tumours of the head, but there is also early spread to regional lymph nodes, the liver and into the posterior abdominal wall.

Sarcomata. These are a rare cause of neoplasia in the young, but behave substantially like adenocarcinomata.

Ampullary tumours. Strictly speaking these are duct tumours but they only differ from other pancreatic tumours in that general spread is comparatively late.

Islet cell tumours. Functioning endocrine tumours can arise from the beta cells (insulinomata) or from γ cells when they commonly secrete gastrin (Zollinger-Ellison syndrome) or, rarely, a different hormone probably secretin (Werner Morrison syndrome). The former is associated with fulminating peptic ulceration (see Chapter 2) and the latter with profuse watery diarrhoea.

Clinical features

Pain. Adenocarcinomata commonly cause pain which may be similar to that of peptic ulcer but without relief from alkalis.

Posterior invasion is associated with back pain, often relieved by bending forward, and sometimes an attack of acute pancreatitis is the first sign of neoplastic disease.

Jaundice. Obstructive jaundice complicates carcinoma of the head, but may temporarily remit due to tumour sloughing.

Other features. Weight loss and mild diarrhoea (usually without clinically obvious steatorrhoea) are common, as are diabetes mellitus, and anaemia due to chronic blood loss. Sometimes there is overt melaena, and occasionally there is migratory thrombophlebitis, usually involving the leg veins. A fixed palpable mass, hepatomegaly and ascites are ominous indicators of far advanced disease.

Diagnosis

Barium meal is seldom diagnostically abnormal, and abnormalities of the duodenal loop are better seen on hypotonic duodenography. Pancreatic function tests (secretin–pancreozymin or Lundh tests) may confirm the presence of pancreatic exocrine insufficiency, and pancreatic scintiscanning or arteriography may respectively show deficient areas of isotope uptake or vascular abnormalities.[126] Tumours involving the duodenal loop can also be seen by duodenoscopy.

Treatment

None of the sophisticated new diagnostic methods has improved the prognosis of pancreatic cancer and the only variety which can be excised with reasonable hope of cure is ampullary cancer. Radiotherapy and antimitotic drugs are valueless: useful palliation of jaundice can, however, be obtained by cholecystjejunostomy.

Clinical features of islet cell tumours

Insulinomata cause recurrent hypoglycaemia with either recurrent attacks of unconsciousness or slow personality change. Diagnostic tests include the provocation of hypoglycaemia by prolonged fasting, and tolbutamide tolerance testing with the measurement of serum insulin levels. Most tumours are single and benign but a few are either multiple or malignant. Because of the problems of managing recurrent hypoglycaemia a determined attempt should be made to extirpate the tumour. When this is impossible diazoxide a hyperglycaemic non-diuretic thiazide may give useful palliation. Clinical features of Zollinger-Ellison syndrome are considered on p. 14.

CARCINOMA OF THE GALLBLADDER

Aetiology and pathology

Approximately four fifths of all patients with gallbladder cancer have gallstones and it seems likely that the stones play a causal role though the mechanism is unknown.[127] Nevertheless very few (perhaps less than 2 per cent) of all patients with stones develop gallbladder cancer and therefore prophylactic cholecystectomy in the frequent elderly people with symptomless stones seems unjustifiable.

Clinical features

These are usually similar to those of chronic cholecystitis though prominent weight loss or a right upper quadrant mass may indicate the real cause. There is usually early invasion of the surrounding structures; therefore the likelihood of surgical cure is small. Radiotherapy and antimitotic drugs, as in other gut cancers, are valueless.

CARCINOMA OF THE BILE DUCT

This rare tumour usually causes early obstructive jaundice, except when only one of the two hepatic ducts are involved. Jaundice may fluctuate due to tumour necrosis, sloughing and relief of obstruction. The diagnosis should always be considered when at operation a patient is found to have a swollen bile stained liver with a collapsed common bile duct.

GASTROINTESTINAL POLYPOSIS

Polyposes can be conveniently divided into those found diffusely throughout the gut and those localized to a specific segment.

Diffuse varieties[128]

(a) Peutz Jeghers syndrome. Hamartomatous polyps (malformations) are found at all sites in the gut, but most often in the small bowel. They are associated with brown pigmented spots on the lips and buccal mucosa. Clinical features include bleeding and intussusception. The polyps are composed of normal epithelium with a branching stroma derived from the muscularis mucosae. The vast majority are not premalignant and surgical treatment is therefore unjustifiable, but there are now several well documented cases where malignancy has supervened.

(b) Juvenile multiple polyposis.[129] These consist of basically normal epithelium arranged somewhat irregularly and the glands often become cystic, due to retained mucus. These are hamartomatous, like Peutz Jeghers polyps, but malignant change has not been described. Most occur in the large bowel and present as rectal bleeding or as prolapsing lesions. No treatment is required except perhaps by rectal fulguration when lower bowel symptoms are prominent.

(c) Pneumatosis cystoides intestinalis. Multiple gas filled swellings develop in the small intestinal and colonic submucosa. Their cause is unknown but there appears to be an association with obstructive airways disease. They can be distinguished radiologically from familial polyposis by the double contrast shadows presented by the gas filled cysts at barium enema examination.

(d) Cronkhite Canada syndrome. The clinical features of this rare disease are, diarrhoea, atrophy of the nails and alopecia. The polyps are due to cystic change in a mucosa with atrophy and secondary inflammatory abnormalities.

Localized polyposis

Stomach. Gastric adenomatous polyps, whether single or multiple are rare. Multiple polyposis is almost certainly premalignant, but single polyps may well remain benign. They are often found incidentally, but may cause haemorrhage. Because of doubts about prognosis they are probably best removed.

Small intestine. Solitary adenomatous, and multiple lymphomatous polyps as a feature of lymphosarcoma, occur rarely. Benign lymphoid polyps also occur, usually in the young and usually localized to the terminal ileum.

FAMILIAL ADENOMATOUS POLYPOSIS COLI

Pathology

Multiple adenomatous polyps develop usually after puberty and histologically can be distinguished from the cystic lesions of juvenile polyposis which develop earlier in life. The condition is inherited as a Mendelian dominant and is often associated with other benign tumours such as fibromata and osteomata (Gardner's syndrome).[130]

Clinical features

Symptoms of diarrhoea and rectal bleeding usually occur in adult life and point strongly towards malignant transformation. If untreated most, if not all, patients with the disease will ultimately develop malignant change.

Diagnosis

The sigmoidoscopic and radiological appearances are characteristic.

Treatment

Once the diagnosis is made then prophylactic colonic excision is essential. Ileorectal anastomosis avoids the need for ileostomy but has the disadvantage of leaving a segment prone to malignant change. This area is easily inspected but the risk of malignant change is so high—perhaps 50 per cent or more that complete large bowel excision is probably preferable.

Since the condition is inherited as a Mendelian dominant thorough family study is essential. It must also be remembered that polyps may not develop until adolescence or early adult life. Children of affected parents should therefore be examined at the age of 17–18. Prior to this age the risk of malignancy, even if polyps are present, is negligible, and it seems right therefore to defer examination and treatment until this age.

Solitary adenomatous polyps

Such lesions are often discovered incidentally but should then be removed surgically as they are probably premalignant. The condition is not, however, an inherited one. Occasionally tumours grow to a large size and assume a villous configuration and if sited in the rectum can cause severe water and electrolyte (especially potassium) deficiency.

Metaplastic polyps

These can be single or multiple—but not in such large numbers as familial adenomatous polyps; they are not premalignant, and represent minor mucosal overgrowths usually with some glandular dilatation. They are commonly seen sigmoidoscopically as small flat mucosal projections.

Chapter 12

INFECTIVE DIARRHOEA

GASTROENTERITIS DUE TO PATHOGENIC *ESCHERCHIA COLI*

Aetiology

This is mainly a disease of young children and is associated with specific serological strains such as 0·55, 111 and 125–128. Infection is not consistently followed by diarrhoea as there is considerable variation in virulence within serotypes.

Clinical features and management

Stools are watery, green and occasionally blood stained. Diarrhoea and associated vomiting may lead to rapid and fatal dehydration or may be comparatively trivial in degree. Persistent vomiting and dehydration are indications for hospital admission and intravenous treatment, especially if associated with convulsions or meningism. A buffered electrolyte solution such as half-strength Hartmanns has much to commend it, especially when dehydration is associated with hypernatraemia.

Antibiotics have no place in management, organisms either are resistant to most of those which are commonly used or rapidly become so, due to transference of resistance.[131]

Constipating drugs are also of little value in infants, and the prime need is for adequate fluid and electrolyte replacement combined with scrupulous hygiene in prophylaxis.

SHIGELLA INFECTIONS

Pathology

These non-lactose-fermenting members of the enterobacteriaceae consist of four subgroups and multiple serotypes identifiable by biochemical serological and phage typing characteristics. Infection is due to faulty hygiene but it should be remembered that organisms can survive for many days in a cool dark atmosphere of high relative humidity.

Clinical features

The large bowel inflammatory response leads to the production of frequent loose stools containing flecks of blood. In severe cases both Flexner and Shiga bacilli can cause mucosal sloughing and necrosis, especially in the sigmoid colon and rectum, with severe dehydration, vomiting and fever. Sonne dysentery is the more frequent in Great Britain and is usually milder and afebrile, but this is a poor discriminant point from the other two varieties, since they can also present in mild forms.

Treatment

Mild cases need little more than a liberal fluid intake, but intravenous therapy may be necessary using 4·3 per cent dextrose in 1/5 normal saline in babies and stronger saline solutions in the elderly.

As in *E. coli* diarrhoea, constipating drugs have little value and antibiotics are of limited usefulness. Though many shigellae are initially sensitive to sulphonamides they soon become resistant through transference. In addition spontaneous stool clearance will take place over a period of weeks irrespective of treatment. It therefore seems reasonable to reserve drug treatment for severe disease, oral streptomycin, neomycin and nalidixic acid are suitable drugs, used according to sensitivity patterns.

SALMONELLOSIS

A large proportion of the hundred odd typhoid and 300 to 400 paratyphoid cases reported annually in England and Wales are contracted abroad.

Typhoid

Pathology

Following ingestion bacilli penetrate the small intestinal wall and are carried to the regional lymph tissue and nodes. They then pass through the thoracic duct to the bloodstream and form widespread secondary foci and can spread from the liver into the bile, accounting for positive faecal cultures in 1–2 weeks after infection.

Clinical features

After a 14, or rarely longer, up to 28 day incubation period, the patient develops malaise and fever together with anorexia, vomiting, constipation and sometimes epistaxis. After a week or 10 days, if untreated the characteristic 'peasoup' diarrhoea develops, there may be splenic enlargement, and in about 20 per cent of cases a 'rose spot' rash on the trunk. Diagnosis should be confirmed by blood, faecal and occasionally urine culture. Delay is inevitable if rising titres of flagellar H or somatic O agglutinins are sought. The detection of Vi antibodies is virtually diagnostic (unlike in particular H which may be high and rise non-specifically because of previous TAB injections).

Treatment

Chloramphenicol 500–1000 mg six-hourly (100 mg/kg bodyweight in children) for at least 14 days is probably the best treatment but the combination of sulphamethoxazole and trimethoprim seems to offer an effective alternative. If initial response is poor then steroids (prednisone 15 mg six-hourly for 3 days, tailing off over the next week) can be added.

Complications

Small bowel haemorrhage and perforation occur due to ulceration of Peyer's patches and there may also be arthritis, pneumonia, myocarditis and osteomyelitis.

Carrier state

This becomes more likely with increasing age, and the frequency has risen with the use of antibiotics. Most chronic carriers have positive Vi agglutinins as well as positive stools. Chloramphenicol is an ineffective and dangerous treatment but ampicillin may be useful if given in high doses for 12 weeks, and recent experience with trimethoprim-sulphamethoxazole is encouraging. Where biliary infection is the cause cholecystectomy may be necessary.

Carriers can be debarred from food handling occupations.

Paratyphoid

Infections with *S. paratyphi* A, B and C are similar to but less severe than typhoid and management is similar to that of typhoid.

Other salmonella infections

Most cases of salmonella enteritis not due to *S. typhi* or *paratyphi* are only of mild or moderate severity and disease is self-limiting. Antibiotic treatment is to be discouraged as it can prolong bacterial excretion except when there is (rarely) severe enteric fever. Treatment is then as outlined for *Salmonella typhi*.

MISCELLANEOUS CAUSES OF FOOD POISONING

Preformed bacterial toxins. These are commonly staphylococcal in origin, are heat stable and produce acute diarrhoea. There is no specific treatment.

Food allergy. Eggs, milk and other foods can cause abdominal pain, diarrhoea and skin rashes in sensitive individuals. There is no treatment.

Poisonous foods and chemicals. The best known poisonous foods are fungi such as *Amanita phalloides*, and *A. muscarina*. These cause initial diarrhoea then vascular collapse and sometimes coma. A variety of chemicals including lead, mercury, cadmium and fluoride can also cause abdominal pain and diarrhoea, amongst other symptoms.

VIRUS INFECTIONS

There is some evidence to show that outbreaks of summer diarrhoea may be due to virus infections, for instance with ECHO viruses. Disease is usually self-limiting. Traveller's diarrhoea is commonly ascribed to viruses, but recent evidence suggests that *E. coli* varieties, especially 0.148, may be responsible,[132] at least for some. Simple treatment with constipating drugs should be prescribed. Antibiotics have no place and probably do little more than encourage the growth of resistant varieties of bacteria. Iodochlorhydroxyquinoline (Enterovioform) is commonly taken as a prophylactic agent There is no good evidence to support this practice and it should be actively discouraged because of the risk of toxic neurological damage, (Subacute myelo-opticoneuropathy).

AMOEBIASIS

Pathology

Amoebae with quadrinucleate cysts infesting man can be separated into three main groups: (a) small avirulent *Entamoeba hartmani*; (b) *E. histolytica*-like amoebae which can multiply at temperatures below 37°C; (c) true large *E. histolytica*, the only group responsible for tissue invasion.[133]

Amoebae are normally dependent upon bacteria for their growth and only become invasive under certain conditions. These have been shown experimentally to include host avitaminosis, mucosal damage, and the presence of certain bacteria, especially *Clostridium perfringens*. Amoebae normally live in the colon especially the caecum and can remain peaceful commensals over many years. Infective disease develops or is precipitated, for instance, by bacterial dysentery, then amoebae penetrate the mucosa and submucosa, there multiplying to form abscesses which burst into the lumen. Further spread can also then occur by the bloodstream.

Clinical features

Diarrhoea tends to be mild but blood and mucus are usually present and symptoms are associated with malaise and mild fever. Spontaneous resolution may then occur after several weeks with or without recurrent disease later. However, even mild cases may develop hepatic and other complications.

Complications—these arise by bloodstream or direct spread and include liver abscesses, and abscesses elsewhere such as the brain and lungs. Liver abscesses may spread locally to penetrate the diaphragm, and gut lesions can coalesce to form an amoeboma, usually caecal in site, a hard mass easily mistaken for carcinoma. Symptoms may develop many years after infection as commensal organisms become virulent—perhaps due to later complicating disease such as bacterial dysentery.

Diagnosis

Microscopy. Microscopic examination of fresh faeces mixed with saline will show active amoebae which contain ingested red cells.

The finding of cysts is harder to interpret; those containing eight nuclei belong to harmless commensals. Cysts with four nuclei may belong to *E. histolytica* to *E. hartmani*, or to *E. histolytica*-like organisms. They can be found in large numbers in carriers as well as in active disease.

Sigmoidoscopy. Discrete irregular ulcers with intervening normal mucosa are classically seen but there may also be more diffuse changes and tiny craters in healing disease. Swabs from ulcer craters, and rectal biopsy revealing intramucosal amoebae will confirm the diagnosis.

Immunological tests. Gel diffusion forms a reasonably simple routine test. Immunofluorescence is also very useful; sera with titres of 1:64 or more strongly suggest recent infection either systemically or locally.

Treatment

Metronidazole in a dose of 800 mg three times daily for 5 days will cure dysentery (100 mg/kg in childhood) whilst 400 mg three times daily for 5 days is effective in liver disease. In dysentery there is remission within 24 hours, in liver abscess there is equally rapid remission of symptoms but the indications for aspiration remain unchanged (these include large or moderately large collections and impending local penetration).[134]

Emetine hydrochloride and chloroquin are also very effective tissue amoebicides when combined, but the risk of toxic complications with emetine injections makes metronidazole preferable. Emetine bismuth iodide (60 mg three times daily for 10 days by mouth) is a reasonably safe and effective alternative to metronidazole for bowel disease: it is relatively non-toxic because poorly absorbed.

Symptomless carriers. If treatment is thought necessary, metronidazole and diloxanide furoate (dose 500 mg three times daily for 10 days) are safe and effective.[135]

GIARDIASIS

Symptoms of diarrhoea and abdominal discomfort are occasionally due to infestion with the protozoan parasite *Giardia lamblia*.

Diagnosis. Organisms can be detected in duodenal juice, and cysts on microscopy of the faeces.

Treatment. Quinacrin 100 mg three times daily for 5–7 days or metronidazole 250 mg t.d.s. for 5–10 days are curative.[136]

BALANTIDIASIS

This is a rare cause of acute or chronic diarrhoea in man.

Diagnosis. Organisms can be detected in faeces or mucosal scrapings.

Treatment. Tetracycline 500 mg four times a day is usually effective.

Chapter 13

INTESTINAL PARASITES

Ancylostomiasis

The hookworms *Ancylostoma duodenale* and *Necator americanus* behave similarly. They live in the small intestine and eggs passed in the stools produce larvae which penetrate the skin and blood vessels, are carried to the lungs where they are trapped, penetrate the alveoli, are carried into the pharynx and swallowed to restart the life cycle in the gut.

Clinical features. These include skin inflammation and lung symptoms as organisms pass through these organs, and diarrhoea and iron deficiency anaemia due to the adult worm's activity. Diagnosis is by finding eggs in the stools. Treatment is given in Table 26.

Ascariasis

Ascaris lumbricoides, the roundworm, lives in the small intestine. Ova are spread by faecal–oral contact, larvae hatch in the small bowel, penetrate the intestinal wall and blood vessels and, like hookworms, cross the alveolar walls and travel up to the pharynx and thence again to the small bowel.

Clinical features. Haemoptysis with eosinophilia and signs of lung inflammation coincide with alveolar affection (Loeffler's syndrome). Adult worms only cause symptoms in heavy infestions when entangled masses can result in intestinal obstruction or when worms block the pancreatobiliary ducts.

Diagnosis is by finding worms in the faeces or occasionally if one is vomited. Treatment for the adult phase is given in Table 26.

Table 26 Treatment for helminthic infections

Ancylostomiasis (hookworm)	Bephenium hydroxynaphthoate (5 g on three successive mornings)	Children, proportional dosage
	Tetrachloroethylene (4 ml in the morning)	Children 0·1 mg/kg
Ascariasis (roundworm)	Piperazine citrate or adipate (150 mg/kg maximum 4 g)	(Simultaneous purgation is advisable)
Fascioliasis (liver fluke)	Bithional (30–40 mg/kg orally on alternate days for 10 doses)	
	Emetine (65 mg daily by injection for 10 days)	
Oxyuriasis (threadworm)	Piperazine citrate or adipate (75 mg/kg daily for 1 week)	
	Viprynium embonate (5 mg/kg one dose, can be repeated after 1 week)	
Schistosomiasis (bilharzia)	Niridazole (12·5 mg/kg twice daily for 7–10 days)	
Strongyloides and trichuris	Thiabendazole (25 mg/kg twice daily for 3 days)	
Taeniasis (tapeworm)	Niclosamide (2 g single dose)	
	Dichlorophen (6 g on each of 2 successive days)	
Trichinosis	Thiabendazole (25 mg/kg daily for 2–3 days)	

Fascioliasis

The liver fluke, *Fasciola hepatica*, has a complicated life cycle, normally involving sheep and snails, and is an accidental parasite of man through ingestion of encysted metacercariae. These mature in the intestine and the larvae penetrate the intestinal wall and migrate to the liver. Infection is well documented as occurring after eating infected watercress.

Clinical features. These include fever, abdominal pain, hepatic tenderness and enlargement with eosinophilia and, occasionally cholecystitis and bile duct obstruction. These features coupled with finding ova in the stool are diagnostic. Treatment could be more satisfactory: recommended methods are given in Table 26.

The life cycle and treatment of *Clonorchis sinensis*, a fluke living in the adult phase in the biliary tree, is essentially similar. It is a cause of obstructive jaundice in tropical areas.

Oxyuriasis

The threadworm, *Oxyuris vermicularis*, is the only common cause of helminthic infection in temperate climates. Adult worms live in the right colon, but the females travel to the rectum to deposit their eggs. Oral ingestion of the eggs is followed by recommencement of the life cycle in the bowel.

Clinical features. Intense perirectal itching due to the activities of the adult females is the only symptom.

Ova deposited on peri-anal skin can be recovered and examined by, for instance, applying cellulose tape and sticking this to a microscope slide. Adult worms can also be detected in the faeces.

Treatment is given in Table 26. Repeated dosage at, or, for one week is needed to kill maturing ova as they hatch in the bowel.

Schistosomiasis

These parasites are responsible for generalized ill health in tropical areas. *Schistosoma mansoni* and *Schistosoma japonicum* cause intestinal disease and *Schistosoma haematobium* (usually) bladder disease. Adult worms live in pairs in the mesenteric or vesical veins and the eggs (which have a spine) penetrate the bowel or bladder wall, when voided hatch into miracidia which infect water snails from which cercarial larvae emerge and penetrate the human skin, enter the blood vessels, and finally reach the abdominal veins.

Clinical features. Skin penetration is associated with itching, urticarial rashes and eosinophilia, passage through the lungs can give rise to pulmonary symptoms. Intestinal varieties cause diarrhoea and abdominal pain with occasionally the passage of blood and mucus. Eggs also become trapped in the portal veins and obstruction, cirrhosis and hepatomegaly ensue. Eggs can be found in faeces and urine, and sigmoidoscopy may reveal groups of small yellow elevated nodules. Rectal biopsy shows submucosal ovae and is an excellent diagnostic method.

Treatment[137,138] detailed in Table 26 is only effective if given in the early stages. It causes electrocardiographic changes and sometimes angina and (more often) nausea and anorexia. The cardiac side effects make bed rest advisable. Antimony preparations are much more toxic though they also give good results.

Strongyloidiasis

This tiny nematode has a similar life cycle to the roundworm, except that larvae can hatch and penetrate the intestinal wall without the eggs leaving the gut.

Clinical features. These include itching with skin penetration, lung symptoms with transalveolar migration and diarrhoea, which may be mild or severe with rectal bleeding and even malabsorption. Larvae are easily found in the stools.

Treatment with thiabendazole (Table 26) is very effective.

Trichuriasis

These small worms live in the colon and seldom cause symptoms except mild diarrhoea. Treatment is the same as for *Strongyloides* (Table 26).

Taeniasis

Taenia solium (pork tape worm), *Taenia saginata* (beef tape worm) and *Diphyllobothrium latum* (fish tape worm) are hermaphroditic ribbon-like segmented worms with a hooked head (scolex) and multiple segments (proglottides) containing the ovae. The adult phase in man is followed by infection of the intermediate host with the cercarial stage. The encysted cercariae are eaten in infected meat and if poorly cooked will survive to form adult worms.

Clinical features. These are commonly abdominal pain and weight loss, and, with the fish tapeworm, megaloblastic anaemia due to competition for vitamin B_{12}. Infection is frequently symptomless, mature segments being recognized in the stools—the usual diagnostic method.

Niclosamide is safe and effective, as is dichlorophen (Table 26) and these are probably preferable to mepacrine. It is important in treatment to expel the scolex otherwise regrowth will occur.

Trichinosis

This disease is acquired by eating pork containing cysts of *Trichinella spiralis*. Young worms are liberated in the gut when the cysts are digested, live temporarily in the small intestine where the females are fertilized, migrate through the gut wall and produce the larvae which enter the lymphatics and blood vessels and are carried throughout the body, encysting in the muscles.

Clinical features. Abdominal pain, vomiting and diarrhoea occur during intestinal invasion and generalized allergic manifestations and sometimes death during parasitic migration in the body. After encystment symptoms disappear.

Allergic symptoms may require steroid treatment; thiabendazole may also be helpful.

Chapter 14

JAUNDICE AND HEPATIC FUNCTION

Liver function tests

The value of many so-called liver function tests is limited and those of practical usefulness are few.

Serum bilirubin. This is a valuable guide to progress, and separation into conjugated and unconjugated varieties can be helpful in diagnosing congenital jaundices.

Alkaline phosphatase. Though classically clearly raised in obstructive jaundice and metastatic disease, and only slightly so in hepatocellular damage there is in practice a considerable overlap. Distinctions are further blurred by the existence of isozymes mainly from liver and bone, but also from intestine and placenta. Concurrent 5'-nucleotidase estimation (derived from liver) is useful in separating liver and bone as sources of alkaline phosphatases.

Aminotransferases. High levels of enzymes such as the serum glutamyl pyruvic transferase (S.G.P.T.) are valuable means of diagnosing active liver disease in acute or chronic active hepatitis.

Protein electrophoresis. This should replace cruder but simpler flocculation and turbidimetric tests. Total serum albumen is a valuable prognostic feature in cirrhosis, and differential globulin measurements may help by distinguishing more diffuse hyperglobulinaemia in cirrhosis from raised gamma-globulin concentrations in chronic active hepatitis.[139]

Bromsulphthalein (B.S.P.) test. Reduced excretion is a sensitive general test in anicteric patients, but useless in jaundice except if recirculation of the Dubin Johnson type is suspected. It is simple but occasional severe anaphylactic reactions have been recorded. (See Chapter 21 for technique.)

JAUNDICE

Pathogenesis. The usual classification into haemolytic, hepatocellular and obstructive varieties though helpful tends to oversimplify the problem. Many problems of jaundice present mixed pictures, particularly of hepatocellular and obstructive jaundice. Furthermore the pathway of bilirubin metabolism is considerably more complex than a simple three stage classification would suggest (Fig. 3).[140]

Pigment overload. The commonest cause is haemolysis, and this can be recognized easily by the combination of mild jaundice anaemia and the almost complete absence of bilirubin from the urine. Further investigations such as reticulocyte count and

Pathway	Abnormality (examples)
Haemoglobin and other haem pigments	Pigment overload—haemolysis, porphyria, shunt hyperbilirubinaemia
↓ Bilirubin (albumen bound)	Drug competition—salicylate, sulphonamide
Transport into liver cells (carrier proteins)	Drug inhibition—flavaspidic acid
↓ Glucuronide conjugation (smooth endoplasmic reticulum)	Absence—Crigler Najjar Impairment—Gilbert, neonatal Competitive inhibition—novobiocin Facilitation—enzyme induction—barbiturates
Excretion (active transport)	Cholestasis Drugs—sensitivity and other mechanisms Congenital defect, Dubin-Johnson syndrome
↓	Also: (a) diffuse hepatocellular damage as in cirrhosis and hepatitis (b) duct obstruction, stone, neoplasm etc

Fig. 3 Disorders of bilirubin metabolism

Coomb's test will be needed to reach a final diagnosis, though it should be remembered that gallstones commonly complicate acholuric jaundice.

Drug competiton for albumen binding sites and drug inhibition of transport into cells. The former is of significance in neonatal life when sulphonamides or salicylates are capable of potentiating kernicterus by preventing bilirubin binding. Drug inhibition of bilirubin transport into cells is of little practical interest now that male fern, which contains flavaspidic acid, is seldom used in treating helminthic disease.

Failure of glucuronide conjugation. This is of particular importance in infancy since hepatic conjugation activity is underdeveloped and there is a risk with pigment overload (commonly in Rhesus incompatibility) of kernicterus and severe brain damage. In addition there are rare cases of congenital severe or mild glucuronyl transferase deficiency Crigler Najjar and Gilbert's disease. Treatment with an enzyme inducing agent, such as phenobarbitone, will lower neontal serum bilirubin levels and is probably of some value in congenital deficiencies[141] but not complete absence of glucuronyl transferase activity.

Failure of excretion into bile canaliculi. The Dubin Johnson syndrome is a congenital example but clinically the important problems are cholestatic drug jaundice, and cholestatic varieties of diffuse liver disease such as hepatitis.

Diffuse hepatocelluar damage. This results mainly in conjugated hyperbilirubinaemia, defective bilirubin excretion being more prominent than abnormalities of bilirubin uptake and conjugation, which are usually slight.

Obstructive jaundice. Features of pale stools and dark urine containing conjugated bilirubin are usually prominent, but the differentiation from hepatocellular damage may be difficult. Obstructive jaundice is considered in more detail on page 162.

Differential diagnosis of jaundice in the newborn

(a) 'Physiological' jaundice of the newborn. This is almost universal, but is accentuated in premature infants and where there is pigment overload due to haemolytic disease. If serum bilirubin concentrations rise above 20 mg per cent there is a strong risk of brain damage due to kernicterus and exchange

transfusion is needed to prevent this. The administration of phenobarbitone (50 to 150 mg daily) to mothers in whom early induction of labour is planned and who have rhesus incompatibility may be helpful in lowering the risk of kernicterus by inducing earlier glucuronyl transferase activity. The same may also be said for phenobarbitone administration to the infant itself.
(b) Congenital defective conjugation (see Crigler Najjar disease).
(c) Primary hepatitis. This uncommon disease is associated with conjugated and unconjugated bilirubin accumulation in the blood. The characteristic histological features on liver biopsy are multinucleate giant cells. The cause is unknown: it can progress to cirrhosis.
(d) Other causes of hepatocellular damage. Cytomegalovirus, herpes simplex and toxoplasma infections can all occasionally cause hepatitis. Congenital syphilis should never be found now that serological testing is a pregnancy routine. Galactosaemia is a cause of prolonged neonatal jaundice. The associated galactosuria is diagnostic. It can also progress to cirrhosis.
(e) Bile duct atresia. Jaundice which is obstructive in type increases steadily from birth. Differential diagnosis from primary hepatitis may be hard, but high serum alkaline phosphatase suggests obstruction and high transaminases are in favour of inflammation. Surgical exploration should always be undertaken as the atresia may be only partial.

Congenital Hyperbilirubinaemias

Unconjugated varieties

Gilbert's disease. This is the commonest variety, is mild (serum bilirubin 1–3 mg per cent) and is often only found incidentally, or is associated with flatulent dyspepsia. The disease appears to be due to a combination of low grade haemolysis, defective uptake into the liver cell and reduced glucuronyl transferase activity. No treatment is usually needed though symptoms may be improved by liver enzyme induction with phenobarbitone.[141]

Crigler Najjar disease. In the severe variety there is complete absence of glucuronyl transferase activity, severe neonatal jaundice, bilirubin 20 mg per cent or more, and kernicterus. In the milder variety serum bilirubin levels tend to be less high, about 10 mg per cent. These can be lowered by giving an enzyme inducing agent such as phenobarbitone or dicophane, which may result in clinical improvement.

Conjugated variety

Dubin Johnson syndrome. Serum bilirubin is usually between 2 and 7 mg per cent and symptoms are minimal or non-existent. Characteristic features are the presence of a brown pigment in liver cells, giving biopsies a diagnostic chocolate brown colour and abnormal bromsulphthalein (B.S.P.) metabolism. Clearance by the liver is normal at one hour but after 2 to 3 hours circulating levels are found to have risen due to recirculation of conjugated B.S.P. No treatment is available or needed.

Rotor syndrome. This a rare variety of conjugated hyperbilirubinaemia, is seldom severe and the cause is not understood.

Differential diagnosis of jaundice in adult life

(a) Haemolysis and congenital hyperbilirubinaemias. Neither of these usually present diagnostic problems. Difficulties commonly arise in distinguishing hepatocellular damage in cirrhosis and hepatitis, from large duct obstruction and particularly in separating cholestatic liver damage from duct obstruction.
(b) Hepatitis. Serum transaminase levels are usually high but alkaline phosphatase levels are only slightly raised if at all, though they can be markedly raised in cholestatic hepatitis. A contact history, transfusion, or injections should also suggest hepatitis. In difficult cases liver biopsy may be needed.
(c) Cirrhosis. Stigmata of chronic liver disease should be sought (Chapter 16). Liver biopsy will usually give confirmatory evidence.
(d) Cholestatic varieties of jaundice. These may be identical clinically with extrahepatic obstructive jaundice and any drug history may be difficult or impossible to elicit. Liver biopsy may show features of bile accumulation with ductular plugging, and transient blood eosinophilia suggests a sensitivity jaundice—for instance due to chlorpromazine.
(e) Extrahepatic obstruction. This is considered on page 162.

Drug Jaundice

The types of drug jaundice commonly recognized and the more frequent causes are given in Table 27.[142]

Haemolysis, conjugation defects and competitive excretion. These are uncommon and are of more physiopathological than clinical interest.

Table 27 Causes of drug jaundice

Specific defects	
Haemolytic	Phenacetin (rare)
Conjugation defect	Novobiocin (dose dependent, good outlook)
Competitive excretion	Cholecystographic media (dose dependent, good outlook)
Cholestatic steroid	Methyl testosterone, norethandrolone and similar drugs (relatively common problem, outlook good)
Cholestatic sensitivity	Phenothiazines of all types (relatively common problem, jaundice can be prolonged, outlook good)
General reactions	
Hepatitic	Iproniazid, phenelzine and similar drugs, halothane (repeated exposure), isoniazid (rarely), methyl dopa (rarely)
Hepatotoxins	Carbon tetrachloride, tetracyclines (avoid large doses especially in pregnancy), paracetamol
Hypersensitivity	Para-aminosalicylate or other anti-tuberculous drugs (may only be cholestatic), erythromycin (estolate only)

Cholestatic reactions

(a) Steroid (non-sensitivity) type. C_{17} substituted testosterones such as norethandrolone can cause a cholestatic reaction, similar to that occasionally described late in pregnancy, and are responsible for the rare instances of oral contraceptive jaundice described especially (and for reasons unknown) in Scandinavia and Chile. Histological changes include bile canicular plugging without inflammation, jaundice is usually mild and recovery is prompt when the drugs are withdrawn.

(b) Sensitivity. Bile duct plugging is associated with a mononuclear cell reaction and evidence of general hypersensitivity such as fever, itching and eosinophilia at the outset. Jaundice is often prolonged, and can occur at any time during treatment. Liver biopsy should make the diagnosis but confusion with biliary obstruction is not uncommon.

Hepatitis

Acute hepatic necrosis, which is usually severe, and is indistinguishable from that occurring in viral hepatitis, is a rare complication of monoamine oxidase treatment. It is also a risk of repeated anaesthesia with halothane; previous mild jaundice or unexplained fever with halothane are warning features.

Hepatotoxins

Carbon tetrachloride and paracetamol, and tetracyclines in large doses in pregnancy are hepatotoxic. Effects are dose related and the picture is that of acute hepatic necrosis.

Hypersensitivity

Generalized evidence of hypersensitivity, with liver damage as a minor component, is an occasional complication of treatment with phenindione, para-aminosalicylic acid, phenytoin, erythromycin and sulphonamides amongst others.

Antibody tests

Antinuclear factor, smooth muscle and antimitochondrial antibodies. These have varying diagnostic usefulness in separating cirrhotic and other liver disease (Table 28). None are organ or disease specific, thus antimitochondrial antibodies are detected using rat kidney rather than liver, and antinuclear factor, though frequently present in chronic active hepatitis, does not denote that the patient has systemic lupus erythematosus.

Alpha 2 foetoprotein. This globulin normally disappears from the circulation at the end of foetal life but reappears in a half to

Table 28 Serum antibodies in chronic liver disease and large duct obstruction[144]

	Percentage incidence		
	Anti-nuclear	Anti-smooth muscle	Anti-mitochondrial
Chronic active hepatitis	56	67	23
Primary biliary cirrhosis	31	50	94
Cryptogenic cirrhosis	16	28	25
Alcoholic cirrhosis	7	0	0
Large duct obstruction	0	0	3

four fifths of those with primary liver cancer (and also in a few with teratoblastoma) and if present is of considerable diagnostic value.

Australia (hepatitis associated) antigen. This is found transiently in acute serum hepatitis (see Chapter 15), occasionally in chronic active hepatitis, and sometimes in Down's syndrome, leprosy and polyarteritis.

LIVER ENLARGEMENT

If the liver is palpable below the costal margin the first task is to determine whether this represents true enlargement. The organ is always palpable in infants, can be frequently felt up to 3 cm below the costal margin on deep inspiration in adults, and can be normal even when palpable on expiration if the patient has depressed diaphragms due to lung disease. Liver dullness usually starts in the fifth intercostal space, and if percussed at a lower level indicates overflated lungs.

Assessment of true size can often be aided by straight abdominal X-ray though this is usually of greater value in determining if the spleen is enlarged as well. After assessing true size, the consistency, regularity and tenderness of the liver must be determined and causes of abnormality considered (Table 29). A hard irregular liver commonly indicates tumour or cirrhosis and a soft or firm tender liver is usually due to hepatitis, cardiac failure or liver abscess, though rapid carcinomatous enlargement can also be tender.

Table 29 Causes of liver enlargement

Anatomical variation	Riedel's lobe, low diaphragm with chronic lung disease
Cirrhosis and inflammation	Cirrhoses of all types, schistosomiasis, hepatitis
Cysts and abscesses	Hydatid disease, polycystic liver, pyogenic and amoebic abscesses
Metabolic disease	Amyloidosis, galactosaemia, glycogen storage disease, lipoidoses, fatty liver
Haematological disease	Leukaemias and lymphomata
Tumours	Primary and secondary carcinoma
Venous and biliary congestion	Heart failure, hepatic vein occlusion, extra- and intrahepatic biliary obstruction

Apart from direct assessment of the liver itself, a search should be made for local or systemic marks of liver disease, such as gallbladder enlargement in obstructive jaundice and spider naevi in cirrhosis. Full physical examination may also reveal a systemic disease of which hepatomegaly is itself only a marker, such as a breast or bronchial tumour.

In addition to biochemical tests of liver function, scintiscanning and biopsy may be necessary to reach a definitive diagnosis.

Scintiscanning

Certain radio-isotopes such as ^{198}Au and ^{99}Tc colloid are selectively taken up by the Kupffer cells and the regular distribution of the gamma irradiation emitted allows the detection of filling defects due to tumours and abscesses, the limit of resolution being approximately 2–5 cm. Isotope uptake tends to be poor and is occasionally irregular in cirrhosis, and there is often high uptake in the spleen. The number of normal anatomical variants on scans can make interpretation difficult, but the technique is in general a valuable diagnostic method.

Liver biopsy

The main indications for this procedure, discussed in more detail in Chapter 16 are the differential diagnosis of hepatomegaly, jaundice and of obscure generalized illnesses where, for instance amyloidosis, tuberculosis, sarcoidosis and reticuloses are suspected. Biopsy is a relatively simple technique but should not be undertaken lightly. It should not be attempted at all in patients with haemorrhagic defects or whose co-operation is doubtful and there are risks of biliary peritonitis and bleeding in patients with severe jaundice. (See Chapter 21 for technique.)

Apart from routine staining for cellular structure, reticulin pattern and iron content, the naked eye appearance of the biopsy may indicate the diagnosis. A fragmented specimen obtained with difficulty may be due to cirrhosis, deep chocolate brown colouring is characteristic of the congenital hyperbilirubinaemia of the Dubin Johnson syndrome, and malignant deposits give rise to scattered pale areas in the specimen.

Chapter 15

HEPATITIS

ACUTE HEPATITIS

Inflammatory disease of the liver varies in duration, cause (Table 30), intensity and pattern and within a continuous spectrum three varieties are discernible.

(a) Hepatic necrosis. This may be so severe that virtually all hepatocytes are lost, and there is collapse of the remaining normal liver architecture. The usual lesion is a centrilobular necrosis with inflammatory cell infiltration.

Table 30 Causes of acute hepatitis

Viral	Long incubation (infective I.H.), short incubation (serum S.H.), glandular fever syndromes
Bacterial	Leptospirosis
Drug induced	(see Table 27)
Childhood	Giant cell hepatitis, congenital toxoplasmasis associated with viral disease, coxsackie, rubella etc
Tropical jaundice	Yellow fever

(b) Anicteric hepatitis. Damage is so slight that there is no jaundice and abnormality is detected because of raised serum transaminases acting as a marker for minimal cell damage.

(c) Cholestatic hepatitis. Jaundice is both prominent and pro-prolonged, and confusion with extrahepatic obstructive varieties may result. Histologically the liver shows a predominant portal tract lesion with canalicular obstruction by bile plugs.

INFECTIOUS HEPATITIS

Pathology and aetiology

This is due to infection with the virus of short incubation (30 day) infective hepatitis (I.H. virus) or long incubation (90 day) serum hepatitis (S.H. virus), the former being chiefly spread by the faecal–oral route and the latter by parenteral contact with blood or blood products infected by a disease carrier. There is no cross immunity between these two infections, and a further distinction is that infective hepatitis tends to be uncommon after young adult life whereas serum hepatitis can occur at any age.

Hepatitis associated antigen (H.A.A. or Australia antigen)[143]

This antigen, first detected in the serum of an Australian aborigine can frequently be found in the serum in the early stages of serum (long incubation period) hepatitis by immunodiffusion and complement fixation techniques. Precise incidence figures are hard to give for it may only be present transiently. It is also frequently found in children with mongolism (who are prone to hepatitis) and occasionally in chronic active hepatitis. The precise nature of H.A.A. is uncertain but blood which contains it will transmit hepatitis, and virus-like particles can be detected by electron microscopy.

Clinical features

After a prodromal period of general malaise, patients develop severe anorexia, nausea and vomiting and occasionally diarrhoea. Fever, right upper abdominal pain and skin irritation are also common. Jaundice may be mild or severe, and bilirubin is detectable in the urine as it is still predominantly conjugated despite the liver inflammation. In some patients cholestasis is so prominent that the clinical picture mimics that of extrahepatic portal obstruction with clay coloured stools and high serum alkaline phosphatase.

The syndrome of fulminant hepatic failure with massive necrosis is relatively uncommon. Basic features, which include mental confusion leading rapidly to coma with associated biochemical and haematological disturbances, are discussed on page 152.

Diagnosis

Jaundice with prominent anorexia and grossly raised serum transaminase levels due to enzyme release by the damaged liver is highly suggestive of infectious hepatitis. In doubtful cases, such as with prominent cholestasis, liver biopsy may be necessary to establish a diagnosis, though this is risky in patients with severe jaundice and coagulation problems. Laparotomy can exacerbate liver cell necrosis and nothing is lost, even in obstructive jaundice, by two or three weeks delay whilst the diagnosis is clarified. In cholestatic disease temporary steroid 'whitewash' may suggest the diagnosis in difficult cases.

Treatment

None is necessary in mild self-limiting disease, the usual variety (though mental depression and raised serum transaminase levels may persist for months).

Bed rest. There is no evidence that variations in activity affect the prognosis, and patients should only rest in bed for as long as general ill health dictates.

Diet. A fat free diet is traditional, but has nothing to commend it beyond the fact that the anorexia of hepatitis is usually combined with a strong aversion to fatty foods. Patients should be encouraged to take a reasonably varied diet but restriction of protein intake and carbohydrate supplementation may be needed if there is massive necrosis.

Steroids. Though corticosteroid drugs may accelerate remission of the jaundice there is no evidence that they alter the ultimate prognosis. They should not normally be prescribed.[146]

Management of fulminant hepatic failure. This is discussed on page 162.

Infectious mononucleosis

Mild jaundice associated with a minor degree of hepatocellular necrosis is common in typical (Paul-Bunnell positive) or atypical (Paul-Bunnell negative) glandular fever.

LEPTOSPIROSIS (WEIL'S DISEASE)

Leptospiral infection, usually with *L. icterohaemorrhagicae*, but occasionally with *L. canicola* and other varieties is acquired through contact, direct or indirect, with rats which excrete the organisms in their urine.

Seven to fourteen days after infection the patient develops an acute illness with fever, severe malaise, backache, muscle pains, and conjunctival suffusion. After several days jaundice, hypotension, oliguric renal failure and leptospiral meningitis may develop together with subcutaneous and subconjunctival haemorrhages. Death is usually due to renal failure but most patients recover uneventfully, especially those with minimal or no jaundice.

The diagnosis is usually confirmed retrospectively by the finding of rising serum agglutinin titres, but organisms can sometimes be found in the blood by dark ground illumination and can occasionally be cultured from blood, and urine after 2 to 3 weeks. Between ten and several hundred lymphocytic cells per mm^3 can be found in the cerebrospinal fluid in most cases of Weil's disease (even without meningitis).

Treatment

Penicillin in large doses (10 mega units daily) is effective in early cases; other antibiotics have proved disappointing.

Drug induced hepatitis: This is considered on page 123.

Childhood hepatitis: See page 121.

Tropical jaundice

Yellow fever: this viral infection carried by the mosquito *Aedes aegypti* causes acute hepatic necrosis. There is no specific treatment. Jaundice in malarial blackwater fever is due to intense haemolysis.

CHRONIC ACTIVE HEPATITIS

Chronic active liver disease as evidenced by mild jaundice, raised serum transaminases and liver biopsy findings of periportal inflammatory change may occur on its own or in association with other disease such as ulcerative colitis, fibrosing alveolitis, and Sjögren's syndrome.

Aetiology

The associations noted with other diseases, which have been thought to have an auto-immune component, have suggested that chronic active hepatitis may also be auto-immune, an impression strengthened by the finding of hypergammaglobulinaemia, antinuclear factor, smooth muscle antibodies but not liver tissue antibodies and response to steroids. It has also been suggested that cases may sometimes follow acute hepatitis and this is supported by the finding of Australia antigen in up to a quarter of patients.

Pathology

It is usual to divide cases into two classes.

Chronic aggressive hepatitis. Inflammatory cells spread into the liver parenchyma from the portal tracts, there is destruction of the limiting plate of parenchymal cells round the portal tracts, and there is piecemeal necrosis of groups of parenchymal cells which are surrounded by inflammatory cells and invading fibrous tissue.

Chronic persistent hepatitis. Though there is a pronounced portal inflammatory reaction, the changes of parenchymal cell destruction, piecemeal necrosis and fibrous invasion are all absent.

Clinical features

These include hepatomegaly, with or without splenomegaly, jaundice and endocrine disturbances with acne, hirsutism and amenorrhoea (the disease is particularly common in young women). Hypergammaglobulinaemia is associated in most cases with the presence of circulating antibodies to smooth muscle (Table 28). Antinuclear factor and lupus cells are also often found and the disease has been called lupoid hepatitis, though it is distinct from systemic lupus erythematosus.

Treatment and prognosis

Persistent abnormal liver function as evidence by raised transaminases but without liver cell necrosis is of good outlook and such cases of chronic persistent hepatitis seldom need treatment. Those with the progressive liver cell damage of chronic aggressive hepatitis fare badly without treatment and usually die with cirrhosis and hepatocellular failure.

Table 31 Prednisone in chronic active hepatitis, outcome of 6 years' treatment[145]

	Alive	Dead
Treated	19	3
Controls	12	15

Steroid treatment will abolish the biochemical abnormalities and there is now good controlled trial evidence that it will improve the prognosis (Table 31).

Chapter 16

CIRRHOSIS AND OTHER LIVER DISORDERS

CIRRHOSIS

Pathology and aetiology

The diagnosis of cirrhosis is based upon three coexisting histological criteria: (a) evidence of liver cell damage, the severity varying, from non-specific degenerative changes to necrosis, from one part of the liver to another, and from one time to another; (b) hepatic fibrosis; (c) nodular regeneration. In these areas multiplying liver cells are found encapsulated in fibrous tissue which produces nodules of varying size distorting normal liver architecture. Fibrosis without nodular regeneration can be found in a number of non-cirrhotic situations, for instance congenital hepatic fibrosis.

It is conventional to distinguish between macronodular and micronodular disease.

Micronodular portal cirrhosis shows an even distribution of nodules a few millimetres in diameter.

Macronodular cirrhosis by contrast contains nodules which are uneven in size and sometimes very large. It is said to be characteristic of posthepatitic cirrhosis but the justification for this view is poor: macronodular cirrhosis can certainly develop in alcoholics, and the risk of cirrhosis occurring at all after infectious hepatitis is extremely small.

Causes of cirrhosis in adult life are listed in Table 32.

Alcoholism. Cirrhosis develops in a small proportion of heavy drinkers. It is unclear, however, why only a minority progress to cirrhosis although alcoholic fatty liver is a universal finding in heavy drinkers. Predisposition to cirrhosis is likely to be based on a combination of genetic and environmental factors; the contribution of malnourishment is not understood.[147]

Table 32 Causes of cirrhosis

Alcoholism
Cryptogenic (seldom if ever viral hepatitis)
Chronic aggressive hepatitis
Haemochromatosis
Wilson's disease (hepatolenticular degeneration)
Primary and secondary biliary cirrhosis
Hepatic venous congestion and veno-occlusive disease
Fibrocystic disease, galactosaemia, glycogenoses

Viral hepatitis. Progressive liver damage after viral hepatitis is now thought to be extremely uncommon. In the vast majority of patients with hepatitis, especially the ordinary short incubation period infective variety, there is complete recovery of normal liver function. The chances of cirrhosis developing may, however, be greater after serum hepatitis.

Chronic aggressive hepatitis. Progressive inflammatory liver disease can ultimately develop into a nodular cirrhosis.

Haemochromatosis. Iron overload, either (probably) due to congenital predisposition or associated with alcohol intake can develop into a typical portal cirrhosis.

Wilson's disease. The cause of cirrhosis is unknown but it is presumably related to the inherited tendency for copper deposition in the liver and elsewhere.

Primary biliary cirrhosis. The cirrhosis is portal in type and is associated with immunological abnormalities and sensitivity injury to biliary duct tissue.

Associated with other diseases. These, such as, secondary biliary cirrhosis with long standing bile duct obstruction, cardiac cirrhosis, and hepatic venous congestion account only for a very small proportion of all cirrhoses.

Cryptogenic cirrhosis. Once all known causes have been listed there remains a further cryptogenic group of varying size who have no detectable predisposing factor. In the United Kingdom these form as many as half the total cirrhotic group, though the proportion is lower in areas, such as France, where alcoholism is a greater problem.

Clinical Features of Cirrhosis

Cirrhosis is usually diagnosed either incidentally as a result of general medical examination, or else because the patient presents with complications of the disease, bleeding, jaundice, ascites or neurological disturbance. Physical features associated with cirrhosis are shown in Table 33. Palmar erythema and clubbing have been ascribed to a hyperdynamic circulation which is also probably associated with abnormal arteriovenous shunting. Failure of inactivation of oestrogens by conjugation has been suggested as the cause of gynaecomastia and testicular atrophy and also of spider naevi (often found in pregnancy). Mild fever is common, probably due to continuing hepatic necrosis.

General investigations

Normochromic or macrocytic anaemia are common, the latter occurring without folate or vitamin B_{12} deficiency. Liver function tests show varying results with low or normal serum albumen, raised globulin, particularly gamma globulin, normal or slightly raised serum bilirubin and normal or raised serum alkaline phosphatase, and transaminases. If all these liver function tests are normal then increased bromsulphthalein retention is a more sensitive index of liver damage. Straight abdominal X-ray may confirm the presence of splenic enlargement undetected clinically.

Table 33 Physical signs in cirrhosis

Skin	Spider naevi, facial telangiectasia, liver palms, finger clubbing
Abdomen	Liver—unduly small or large, splenomegaly, ascites, collateral veins
Endocrine	Gynaecomastia, loss of body hair, small testes
Neurological	Hepatic flap, disorientation, coma, neuromyelopathy
General	Fever, parotid enlargement and Dupuytren's contracture

Liver biopsy

This should be carried out in all patients with suspected cirrhosis, provided there is no abnormal bleeding tendency and the patient is fit to co-operate during the procedure.

Biopsy is extremely accurate diagnostically, failure being commonly due to obtaining a fragmented specimen without fibrous tissue with a Menghini needle or to chance biopsy of normal liver from a single large nodule. Routine staining should be carried out for hepatic cells (haematoxylin and eosin) fibrous tissue (Van Gieson's stain) and iron (Perl's reagent). Estimation of copper should also be considered. Excessive iron deposition in the liver is not uncommon in ordinary (non-haemochromototic) cirrhosis, so that the finding of moderate excesses of liver iron is hard to interpret in isolation.

Other investigations. These are considered in relation to specific types of cirrhosis.

Complications

Portal hypertension. Obstruction to portal venous return is followed by a rise in pressure in the blocked vein and collateral vessels may develop, particularly around the oesophagus. This problem is considered in more detail in Chapter 17.

Neurological disturbance and jaundice. Deterioration of liver cell function is followed by a variety of neuropsychiatric phenomena and deepening jaundice; these are considered further in Chapter 18.

Ascites and oedema. Deteriorating liver function is also associated with a fall in serum albumen, rise in portal pressure, ascites, sodium retention and oedema. This problem is discussed in Chapter 18.

Other complications

Hepatoma. A fifth of all cirrhotics develop primary liver cancer. This is often multifocal, but may be single. Diagnosis is usually late because local spread produces no symptoms, and these only appear if there is rapid liver enlargement, portal vein obstruction leading to bleeding varices or ascites; or direct spread beyond the liver giving ascites, intraperitoneal bleeding or local bony disease. Isotope scintiscanning may indicate a large focal lesion but it has recently been shown that many cirrhotics with liver cancer have a foetal globulin, α_2-foetoprotein in large amounts in their serum. This is presumably derived from the neoplastic liver cells and is a valuable diagnostic test.

Peptic ulcer. Gastroduodenal ulcer is a frequent concomitant of cirrhosis and is believed to be more common than would be expected by chance, especially after a shunt operation.

Tuberculosis. Debilitated and alcoholic patients are particularly at risk of tuberculosis, especially of the lung and complicating ascites.

Specific Varieties of Cirrhosis

Alcoholic and cryptogenic

Distinctions are few between these two varieties of cirrhosis. Clinically Dupuytren's contracture and parotid enlargement are said to be commoner in the alcoholic variety as are neuropathy, cardiomyopathy and cerebral deterioration, but the cirrhosis itself is indistinguishable apart from the presence of alcoholic hyalin.

The cause of alcoholic cirrhosis is almost as obscure as that of the other variety (the term cryptogenic meaning of hidden cause). Alcohol is metabolized in the liver, and fatty accumulation is an invariable feature of the alcoholic's liver. However, the cause of the change from fatty degeneration to cirrhosis is not understood. An easy explanation is the coincidence of a toxic effect of alcohol with a poor diet, but this case has never been proved, and no dietary lack which predisposes to cirrhosis in man has yet been identified. Similarly no clear genetic predisposing factors have been isolated.

Treatment. None has been shown to alter the prognosis of cryptogenic liver disease and management is essentially that of the complications. The progress of alcoholic cirrhosis can, however, be retarded by abstinence, with, in particular, rapid regression of fatty infiltration, reduction in liver size and loss of hyalin.

Steroids. No overall differences were found in survival in two large groups of cirrhotic patients, one of whom received steroids and the other who did not. Within this overall result women without ascites fared relatively well on steroids (possibly because many had chronic aggressive hepatitis—see Chapter 15), and patients with ascites fared badly on steroids (Table 34).

Prognosis. The overall outlook in cryptogenic cirrhosis, and in alcoholics who continue to drink, is particularly bad and less than 20 per cent are still alive after 5 years.

Postviral hepatitis. Cirrhosis after viral hepatitis (if it occurs) does not differ materially from cryptogenic cirrhosis.

Table 34 Steroid treatment in cirrhosis[149]

	No. studied	Percentage dying		
		Overall	Non-ascitics	Ascitics
Prednisone	169	41	28	78
Control	165	42	37	53

Haemochromatosis

Pathology

In this disease hepatic iron stores are grossly in excess of normal, iron being present in large amounts in hepatic cells, and there is concurrent deposition of iron elsewhere, particularly in the heart, pancreas and testes. Serum iron levels are usually also grossly raised at more than double the normal value of 70 to 150 μg per cent, and there is almost complete saturation of the iron binding capacity of transferrin.

Aetiology

The causes are poorly understood but certainly include genetic predisposition, for both patients and their relatives have abnormally large iron stores. Excessive iron absorption does not seem to be due to secretory factors and an abnormality of intestinal cell function seems most likely. The situation is complex, however, for cirrhotics without haemochromatosis occasionally have large hepatic iron stores as do patients who have had portasystemic shunt procedures. Simple iron overload by diet or transfusion also increases liver stores but this siderosis only rarely seems to be complicated by haemochromatosis.

Clinical features

The disease is seldom found in menstruating women (because of the recurrent iron loss) but can present postmenopausally.

The classical clinical features are liver enlargement, diabetes mellitus (latent or overt), skin pigmentation, impotence and arthritis.

Diagnosis

A high serum iron, saturated iron binding capacity and biopsy evidence of cirrhosis with excess iron stores will ordinarily confirm the diagnosis. In doubtful cases the use of the iron chelating agent diethylenetriamine penta-acetic acid (D.T.P.A.) together with radioactive iron (^{59}Fe) may show evidence of grossly excessive iron stores though overlap with simple alcoholic cirrhosis and shunt patients has been found.[148] In haemosiderosis iron will be found mainly in Kupffer cells rather than parenchymal cells, and there is no cirrhosis.

Treatment

Chelating agents are ineffective and venesection is the only useful method. Each week 500 ml should be removed until excess iron stores have been lost. Complications, diabetic and otherwise, should be treated as necessary.

Wilson's disease (hepatolenticular degeneration)

Pathology

This familial disease is inherited as an autosomal recessive and is associated with abnormally high intestinal copper absorption, near absence of copper carrying protein (caeruloplasmin) from the blood and excessive copper deposition in the tissues, especially liver and brain, and excretion in the urine.

Clinical features

Hepatic. Any of the usual features of cirrhosis may be present but usually only when neurological disease has been obvious for some time.

Neurological. Copper deposition in cerebral extrapyramidal tissues gives rise to softening and cystic change in these areas, clinically manifested as rigidity and coarse tremor affecting large joints. Intellectual deterioration appears at a later stage.

Kayser Fleischer rings. Slit lamp examination will reveal characteristic greenish brown copper deposits on the back of the cornea inside the limbus.

Other changes. Occasionally nail discolouration (azure crescents) and bone disease, (osteomalacic or porotic with osteoarthritis) coexist. Aminoaciduria is also a constant feature.

Diagnosis

Copper retention in the liver and excess in the urine are diagnostic features. Low serum caeruloplasmin levels are also found (but sometimes in other liver disease as well).

Treatment

Administration of the copper binding compound dimethyl-cysteine (D. penicillamine) 20–40 mg/kg daily will slowly over many months produce partial or complete reversal of brain and liver damage by causing increased urinary copper excretion.

As damage is not always reversible there is much to be said for screening relatives by liver biopsy. Low copper diet and oral potassium sulphide (to bind dietary copper) are secondary methods of treatment.

Primary biliary cirrhosis

Pathology and aetiology

Inflammatory change is concentrated in this condition in the pericholangiolar tissue with round cell and plasma cell infiltration and fibrosis spreading from the portal tracts to give cirrhosis. The high frequency of mitochondrial antibodies, which are not tissue specific but are seldom found in other varieties of liver disease (Table 28) or other non-specific inflammatory disease, and the lymphocytic infiltration, strongly suggest an autoimmune process.

Clinical features

These typically consist of mild but progressive jaundice,

obstructive in type, usually in middle aged women. It is associated with hepatosplenomegaly, pruritus, cutaneous xanthomata (associated with hypercholesterolaemia), steatorrhoea and in the late stages osteomalacia.

In the late stages the usual complications of severe cirrhosis often appear also.

Investigations will show the characteristic raised alkaline phosphatase and serum bilirubin of obstructive jaundice with raised α_2 and β-globulins or γ-globulins. The diagnosis is based upon the combination of pericholangiolar cirrhosis with high titre antibodies with lack of evidence of bile duct obstruction.

Treatment

Steroids and immunosuppressives have yet to be shown to be useful. Pruritus will be relieved by cholestyramine (Questran) administration to interrupt the enterohepatic circulation of bile acids—the probable cause of itching.[150] A low fat diet will help the steatorrhoeic diarrhoea and vitamin D supplements may be needed to treat osteomalacia.

Prognosis

Though patients live for several years, death with cirrhotic complications inevitably supervenes.

Other varieties of adult cirrhosis

Secondary biliary cirrhosis (consequent upon bile duct obstruction). This is considered on page 163.

Cardiac cirrhosis. Centrilobular congestion of long standing due to obstruction of venous return, for instance in congestive heart failure or constrictive pericarditis is followed by a perivenous fibrous reaction which can spread into the portal tracts and ultimately result in nodular hyperplasia. Ascites is a common clinical problem and the liver is frequently covered in a thick fibrinous exudate. Mild jaundice, similar to that of passive venous congestion is usually present, but portal hypertension and neuropsychiatric sequelae are rare.

Budd Chiari syndrome (hepatic vein occlusion). This rare condition is usually caused by tumours involving the inferior vena cava and by clotting diseases such as polycythaemia rubra vera. It has also been described following oral contraceptive treatment, and vena caval stricture and web have occasionally been found. In the acute variety there is the sudden onset of abdominal pain, liver enlargement, jaundice and ascites, followed in total occlusion by death with hepatocellular failure. In the chronic form jaundice is an inconstant feature or often absent altogether and portal hypertension with varices and ascites develop as complications. Clinically the liver is large and tender; pressure over it will often fail to fill the jugular veins. Treatment is symptomatic for the complications except that strictures and membranous obstructions to the vena cava can be treated surgically.

Veno-occlusive disease. Obstruction to small hepatic veins with centrizonal fibrosis has been described as a complication of taking *Senecio, Heliotropium* and *Crotolaria* (bush tea) as herbal medicines, often in small children. The disease shows the usual features of an acute or chronic Budd Chiari syndrome and is due to poisoning by pyrrolizidine alkaloids.

Cirrhosis in childhood

As in adults the cause of cirrhosis in childhood is frequently obscure. Wilson's disease (hepatolenticular degeneration), galactosaemia, glycogen storage diseases and veno-occlusive disease can all cause childhood cirrhosis. In addition neonatal giant cell hepatitis can progress to cirrhosis, and biliary atresia to a secondary biliary cirrhosis. Cirrhosis is also an occasional late complication of mucoviscidosis.

OTHER LIVER DISEASE

Infiltrative disease

Amyloidosis. Primary and (more commonly) secondary amyloid may be found in the liver, and can give rise to massive enlargement. Biopsy is diagnostic.

Fatty change. Fatty degeneration is common in chronic alcoholism, where the presence of Mallory's alcoholic hyaline may be a useful diagnostic point. Damage is reversed by abstinence.

Fatty liver is also common in kwashiorkor, a frequent disease in protein-deficient and generally malnourished populations, as well as in any chronic debilitating illness, such as ulcerative colitis and in untreated insulin dependent diabetics—where there may be obvious temporary hepatomegaly.

Lipoidoses. Liver enlargement, and splenomegaly, are common and the lipids typical of the variety can be identified histologically. Lipoidoses do not cause hepatocellular failure.

Galactosaemia. Congenital inability to convert galactose to glucose due to lack of galactose-1-phosphate uridyl transferase causes failure to thrive in infancy with hepatomegaly (due to fatty infiltration and later cirrhosis), aminoaciduria, mental retardation and cataracts. Galactose must be withdrawn early from the diet if changes are to be reversed.

Glycogen storage diseases. In five varieties there is inability to break down glycogen, in one (branching enzyme deficiency) because of abnormal glycogen structure and in four (glucose-6-phosphatase, liver phosphorylase, debranching enzyme and alpha glucosidase deficiencies) because of lack of normal metabolic pathways. Clinical features include gross hepatomegaly, hypoglycaemia, ketosis and retarded growth. There is no specific treatment, hypoglycaemia demands frequent glucose feeds, but otherwise a low carbohydrate diet is desirable.

Granulomatous infiltration. The discovery of scattered hepatic granulomata on liver biopsy is often helpful in diagnosing obscure general illnesses. Commoner causes include tuberculosis, sarcoidosis, brucellosis, fungal disease, histoplasmosis, and schistosomiasis.

Haemosiderosis. Iron deposition in the liver without haemochromatosis occurs after prolonged excessive iron therapy or iron ingestion (as in the Bantu from habitually using iron cooking vessels), following multiple (100 or more) blood transfusions for instance in aplastic anaemia and after portacaval shunt operations.

Iron is concentrated in the Kupffer cells in the portal areas, there is no cirrhosis and serum iron levels are seldom excessive. Haemosiderosis causes no symptoms and attempts to deplete patients by bleeding lead to anaemia but no benefit. The borderlines with haemochromatosis are, however, somewhat blurred because cirrhotics especially those with portosystemic collaterals have excess hepatic iron and occasionally there is diagnostic confusion.

Congenital hepatic fibrosis. In this rare condition normal hepatic lobules are intersected by dense bands of fibrous tissue, and it is not a cirrhosis. Children or young adults present with symptomless liver enlargement, splenomegaly or bleeding oesophageal varices due to associated portal hypertension. The prognosis is good if portal hypertension can be controlled and patients are excellent subjects for portacaval anastomosis. It is often misdiagnosed as juvenile cirrhosis.

Cysts

Polycystic liver. There are multiple cysts, commonly in the liver and kidneys but, unlike renal cysts, the liver cysts, which probably represent intralobular bile duct remnants, seldom cause symptoms, though the liver may be moderately enlarged.

Hydatid cysts. Ova of *Taenia echinococcus* passed in dog faeces will hatch in the intestine if ingested by man and pass through the bowel wall via the portal vein to the liver. There cysts grow and produce daughter cysts to give large masses. These can spread by rupture into the bloodstream or through the diaphragm.

Clinical features. Liver enlargement is usually the first sign of the disease but cyst leakage can cause severe hypersensitivity reactions, fever, or abdominal pain. Calcified cysts are often visible on X-ray, and the Casoni test is a good indicator of the disease, though false positive results can occur. Specially prepared filtered hydatid fluid (0·2 ml) is injected intradermally and evidence of a resulting wheal is sought after 30 minutes.

Treatment. Surgical excision is seldom possible and cysts can usually only be evacuated and attempts made to sterilize the cavity with sclerosing fluid.

Liver abscesses

Abscesses may be due to bacterial or amoebic infection. The clinical features, which are the same, include fever, hepatomegaly often with a raised right diaphragm, leucocytosis and toxaemia. The management of amoebiasis is discussed in Chapter 12.

Multiple pyogenic abscesses commonly arise secondary to portal pyaemia for instance with appendix abscess. However, they can also occur secondary to cholecystitis and cholangitis amongst other diseases.

A single abscess can occur on its own without any apparent predisposing infection, or it can arise in association with intra-abdominal sepsis.

Clinical features. There is usually a swinging fever, leucocytosis and hepatic tenderness, but small and single lesions may cause malaise, normochromic anaemia, weight loss and nothing else. Portal pyaemia and cholangitis are associated with mild jaundice.

Liver scan will usually confirm that there is an hepatic filling defect or defects, but clinical differentiation from subphrenic or perinephric abscess may be well-nigh impossible. Treatment includes broad spectrum antibiotics, such as ampicillin, and drainage by aspiration or preferably exploration.

Chapter 17

PORTAL HYPERTENSION

Hepatic parenchymal cells have two blood supplies, one through the hepatic artery and the other through the portal venous system which is interposed between two sets of capillary vessels, in the intestine and spleen on the one hand, and on the other in the hepatic sinusoids. Obstruction to portal venous flow may occur at two levels, presinusoidally in the portal venous system itself and postsinusoidally in the hepatic venous system. Obstruction may raise portal pressure to double or more the usual level of 3–17 mm of mercury and induces the development of collateral vessels. These are commonly sited: (a) at anastomoses between gastric and oesophageal veins; (b) at spleno-oesophageal and diaphragmatic or peritoneal anastomoses; (c) through the umbilical veins; (d) between the superior surface of the liver and the diaphragm; (e) through the mesenteric and haemorrhoidal veins.

Clinical features

By far the most important clinical collateral vessels are the submucous gastro-oesophageal veins which can dilate enormously and then rupture usually causing massive gastrointestinal bleeding. Umbilical venous dilatation (caput Medusae) can act as a clinical marker for this condition, and there is usually splenic enlargement, though splenomegaly frequently occurs in liver disease without portal hypertension.

Leucopenia and thrombocytopenia are commonly associated with splenomegaly, and any of the usual features of chronic liver disease may be manifest, especially ascites in view of the interrelationships of portal pressure and hypoalbuminaemia in its genesis.

Diagnosis

The most important cause of portal hypertension in Britain and the U.S.A. is cirrhosis, but elsewhere other disease, such as schistosomiasis, assumes greater importance. Nevertheless even in areas where cirrhosis is common it is unwise to assume that varices have caused bleeding. Peptic ulcer is also a common concomitant of liver disease.

Diagnosis depends upon the demonstration of varices either by barium swallow or oesophagoscopy. Of these oesophagoscopy is probably the more accurate as well as the more unpleasant. Dependence upon biochemical tests such as evidence of bromsulphthalein (B.S.P.) retention is unwise because peptic ulcer and liver disease coexist and because B.S.P. may be retained in ulcer bleeding.

Management

The principles are to restore blood volume, to control bleeding and to prevent encephalopathy (consequent upon reduced liver function with hypotension and anoxia and upon sudden gastrointestinal protein loading with the haemorrhage).

Transfusion

Fresh blood may be necessary to help compensate for deficient clotting factors due to liver disease. Vitamin K_1 should also be given (10 mg intramuscularly to control hypoprothrombinaemia).

Control of bleeding

Vasopressin. Initially vasopressin, 20 u in 100 ml of dextrose, should be given over 20 minutes and this can be repeated after 4 hours. It has a splanchic vasoconstrictor action as well as an initial general peripheral vasoconstrictor effect.

Side effects include pallor, hypertension, colic and purgation, which can be useful in clearing the bowel but the drug should if possible be avoided in cardiac disease. Its mesenteric vasoconstrictive effect may also, theoretically, reduce liver blood supply and further impair liver function.

Balloon tamponade

If vasopressin is ineffective then direct pressure on varices with the Sengstaken tube may be tried. The treatment is unpleasant for the triple lumen tube is of wide bore and the inflated oesophageal and gastric balloons prevent normal swallowing, so that pharyngeal secretions have to be aspirated for otherwise there is a risk of spillover lung disease. Liquids can, however, be introduced direct into the stomach through the third lumen. Balloon pressure should be maintained at above variceal pressure, about 40 mmHg, but never for longer than 24–36 hours. Before tamponade is attempted, a decision should be made as to whether the patient is fit for an operation or would withstand further bleeding (which is common on decompression). If not then it is unkind to undertake anything more than terminal care (Fig. 4).

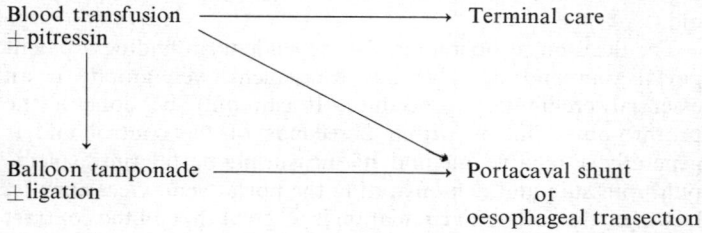

Fig. 4 Management of bleeding oesophageal varices

Hypothermia

Circulation of a water–ethanol mixture at a temperature of 0°C down an oesophageal tube and through a gastric balloon is as effective as balloon tamponade, and as unpleasant. It stops bleeding by inducing local vasoconstriction but recurrence is common.

Early recurrent bleeding

Operation should be undertaken only in those with good liver function. Basic discriminants are the presence or absence of severe jaundice, coma or ascites. Patients free of these complications should be considered for either direct oesophageal surgery or emergency portacaval shunt. The former, by ligation of varices or oesophageal transection is simpler and has the advantage that once bleeding is controlled the pros and cons of portacaval shunting can be compared at leisure.

Late recurrent bleeding and surgery

Long term protection against recurrent bleeding is best provided by portacaval shunt operations. The chances of later neuropsychiatric sequelae are high, however, and must be reduced by selection of patients with probable good liver function. Such evidence is ideally provided if (a) there has been no coma or ascites, (b) there is no jaundice and serum albumen is greater than 3·0 g per cent and (c) the patient is under 50 years old.

The decision to operate is also dependent on finding a patent portal vein and percutaneous transsplenic venography is an essential preliminary procedure. It can only be done if the prothrombin time is within 2 seconds of the control and is generally a reliable method of measuring portal (intrasplenic pulp) pressure and demonstrating the portal vein. Occasionally, however, the collateral circulation is so great that all the contrast medium bypasses a patent vein. Coeliac or superior mesenteric arteriography is a useful alternative in patients who have had a splenectomy.

Portacaval shunting is usually done end-to-side[152] anastomosing the cut portal vein to the vena cava but splenorenal or mesenteric caval shunts (side-to-side) may be the only possible procedure in those with portal vein thrombosis. They divert a smaller proportion of blood and secondary thrombosis is commoner than after portal caval operations.

Results of surgery

The frequency of recurrent bleeding is dramatically reduced after portacaval shunting and decompression would also be expected to prevent ascites formation. However, the operative mortality is between 10 and 15 per cent, overall mortality is high, hepatic encephalopathy is common despite careful selection (Table 35) and haemosiderosis is frequently seen.

Table 35 Emergency treatment for portal hypertension

Operative mortality[154]	No. of patients	Percentage mortality
Emergency procedure	173	31·8
Therapeutic for previous bleed	1244	15·5
Prophylactic operation	137	4·4

Morbidity after prophylactic shunt		Percentage with	
	No. of patients	Recurrent bleed	Complicating encephalopathy
Medical treatment only[153]	73	26	5·5
Prophylactic shunt	68	1·5	25·0

In young patients with good liver function the risks of recurrent bleeding after control of an initial episode are such that there is probably no alternative to operation. But it is doubtful if prophylactic shunting can be justified in those with proven varices but no bleeding.[151] In three trials conducted in the U.S.A. it was found that shunting conferred protection against bleeding but did not reduce the mortality rate.

Chapter 18

ASCITES AND HEPATOCELLULAR FAILURE

ASCITES

The presence of ascites in the absence of a local cause, such as peritoneal tumour or inflammation, or renal and cardiac disease is strongly indicative of advanced hepatocellular failure.

The main factors affecting fluid transfer between the intra and extravascular compartments are the effective colloid osmotic pressure exerted by the serum albumen (intravascular colloid osmotic pressure minus ascitic colloid osmotic pressure–if present) and the effective portal pressure (portal venous pressure minus abdominal hydrostatic pressure).[155]

In cirrhosis (Fig. 5) the effective colloid osmotic pressure is reduced, because serum albumen is low and also often because of the opposing effect of albumen present in ascitic fluid. Secondly portal venous obstruction causes portal hypertension and thirdly any hepatic outflow block leads to lymph loss into the peritoneal cavity.

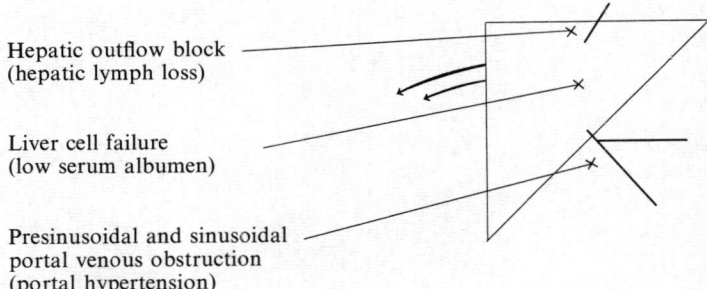

Fig. 5 Causes of hepatic ascites

Fluid balance is further disturbed by avid sodium retention by mechanisms shown in Figure 6 and by water retention secondary to sodium retention and (perhaps) to inappropriate antidiuretic hormone release. There is also failure of cellular conservation mechanisms for potassium.

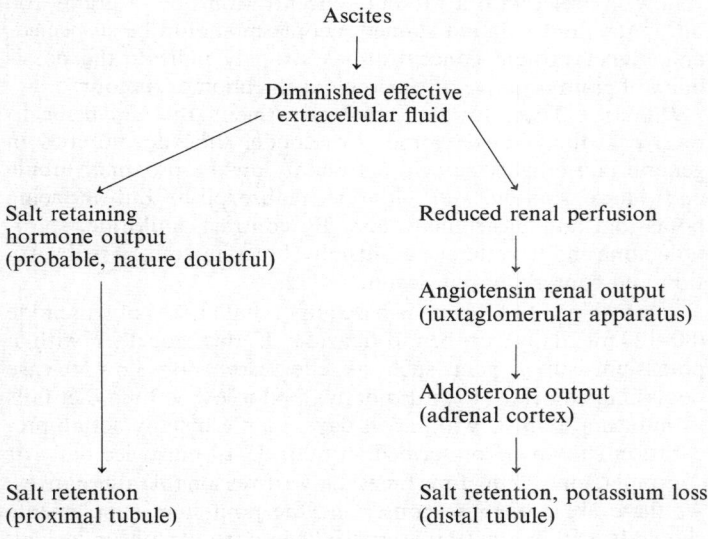

Fig. 6 Causes of salt retention in hepatic ascites

Clinical features

Ascites indicates either that liver disease is severe or that it has been complicated by peritoneal infection, primary carcinoma or hepatic vein occlusion. Apart from the characteristic shifting dullness and fluid thrill, portal vein collaterals secondary to obstruction may be seen radiating from the umbilicus. Hydrothorax (due to free communication between the peritoneal and pleural cavities) is not uncommon and peripheral oedema, if present, is less marked than the ascites.

Management

Paracentesis. Diagnostic tap of 50 ml for examination for evidence of infection or malignancy should be carried out, but larger amounts should only be removed to relieve pain as the tap will exacerbate the tendency to fluid accumulation by removing albumen, and predisposes to hepatic coma. Fluid should be yellowish green with a protein concentration of 1–2 grams/100 ml. If the fluid is blood stained, neoplasm should be suspected, and higher protein concentrations strongly indicate the possibility of gram negative or tuberculous infection or tumour.

Diuretics. These form the main treatment, the aim being to reverse sodium conservation. Frusemide, thiazide diuretics in general and ethacrynic acid act mainly on the proximal tubule and block sodium and chloride reabsorption but inducing potassium and bicarbonate loss. By contrast amiloride, spironolactone and triamterene act distally, blocking sodium reabsorption and conserving potassium.

A sensible initial regime is based upon high doses of frusemide (80–120 mg daily) or bendrofluazide. If this, together with a potassium supplement such as effervescent or slow release potassium chloride (100 mEq daily), and a low sodium diet fails to induce a diuresis within 3–4 days, then a distally acting preparation should be prescribed. Amiloride 10 mg twice daily or spironolactone 25 mg four times daily are reasonable alternatives. As these are potassium conserving the potassium supplements should be withdrawn (this is especially important with amiloride). Triamterene is probably the last choice because it can cause hyperkalaemia and azotaemia.

Sodium restriction. Intake should be reduced to about 20 mEq (450 mg) daily.

Results and complications of diuretic treatment

Most patients respond well to combined diuretic and salt-restrictive treatment.

Hypokalaemia: This is common and is due in part to the effects of proximal tubular diuretics and in part to secondary aldosteronism. Potassium supplements must be given as the chloride as they will not otherwise be retained. The effervescent variety (6·5 mEq per tablet) and slow release type (8 mEq per tablet) are interchangeable. Over vigorous diuretic therapy and ensuing hypokalaemia predispose to hepatic coma.

Resistance to treatment: With or without electrolyte disturbance this implies severe liver disease of poor prognosis.

Hyponatraemia: In isolation this is usually due to sodium loss but relative water retention, serum sodium will be less than 130 mEq/litre. It can be treated by fluid restriction (less than 500 ml daily) mannitol infusion (2 litres of 10 per cent solution intravenously as an osmotic diuretic) or with prednisone (which increases glomerular filtration and water loss).

Combined hyponatraemia, hypokalaemia and azotaemia: This implies severe (and perhaps untreatable) liver disease or over-enthusiastic therapy.

Albumen infusions. These may be effective in inducing a diuresis in refractory patients but are ineffective, expensive and inconvenient for maintenance treatment.

Portacaval shunt. Though portal hypertension and hence ascites may be relieved, neuropsychiatric sequelae are so common due to the severe liver disease that the procedure cannot be recommended.

Prognosis

Sixty per cent of patients with ascites and cirrhosis die within 2 years. The terminal episode usually includes hypotension, oliguria and azotaemia, or hyponatraemia, due in part to reduced renal perfusion. Nothing is gained by trying to treat them.

HEPATOCELLULAR FAILURE

Acute or chronic liver cell failure may be followed by a variety of neuropsychiatric and other sequelae. These include: (a) coma or encephalopathy associated with acute hepatic necrosis or portosystemic encephalopathy, (b) biochemical and haematological disturbances consequent upon liver cell failure, and (c) chronic neuropsychiatric sequelae.

Hepatic encephalopathy

The mechanism by which this is produced is poorly understood but it seems to be due to the accumulation of toxic nitrogenous products in the body. Thus encephalopathy may be precipitated in patients with advanced liver cell failure by excessive protein intake and by ammonium salt ingestion and a reasonable, but not perfect, correlation can be found between the blood ammonium concentration and the development of the syndrome. Ammonia is known to be converted by the liver to urea; however, it is unclear whether ammonia is itself toxic or whether it acts as a marker for other substances, such as secondary amines.

Clinical features

The neurological features of hepatic encephalopathy include drowsiness, confusion, inco-ordination and dyspraxia. Drowsiness may progress rapidly to coma particularly in patients with acute hepatic necrosis—for instance due to drugs. Confusion can lead to inappropriate social behaviour or may be illustrated only by general intellectual deterioration. Inco-ordination is shown by the characteristic flapping tremor of the outstretched hands. Dyspraxia is commonly tested by asking the patient to copy a five pointed star. Foetor hepaticus which has a peculiar sweetish smell is an associated feature of encephalopathy together with a hyperdynamic peripheral circulation.

It is useful to distinguish between precoma and coma associated with acute hepatic necrosis and that associated with chronic liver disease, portosystemic encephalopathy.

Acute hepatic necrosis. Fulminant hepatic failure due to viral or drug hepatitis tends to progress rapidly from confusion to coma. It tends to be difficult or impossible to reverse and is associated with electrolyte imbalance, disturbance of carbohydrate metabolism (hypoglycaemia) and haemostatic failure.

Portosystemic encephalopathy. This is due to overstressing of a chronically damaged liver by products of protein metabolism. It may be precipitated by: (a) dietary protein overload, (b) gastrointestinal bleeding where hypotension may impair hepatic ability to cope with the protein load, (c) electrolyte imbalance in diuretic treatment, (d) infections, (e) portal-systemic bypass either through collateral veins such as oesophageal varices or a portacaval shunt which transfers intestinal venous blood direct to the circulation bypassing the liver, and (f) drugs, such as barbiturates and morphine alkaloids.

Treatment[156]

Protein restriction. All protein should be removed from the diet and as recovery occurs should be added in progressive 20 g per day steps every few days.

Antibiotics. Oral neomycin 1 g every 6 hours is the standard method for reducing nitrogenous metabolism by eliminating gut bacteria.

Laxatives. Constipation should be treated vigorously with enemata and a regular bulk laxative such as magnesium sulphate or lactulose should be administered. Catharsis with lactulose (30–120 ml daily) may have special advantages in that the acid stools produced by bacterial activity in breaking down this synthetic non-absorbed sugar may inhibit ammonia absorption.[158]

General measures. These include vigorous treatment of infections, transfusion in anaemic patients, and the correction of electrolyte imbalances, commonly potassium depletion caused by overenthusiastic thiazide treatment of ascites. Patients are also very sensitive to barbiturate and morphine-like drugs because of the reduced capacity of hepatic detoxicating mechanisms.

Surgery. In resistant cases of portosystemic encephalopathy, especially after technically successful portacaval shunting, colonic exclusion by ileorectal anastomosis has occasionally proved the only method which will reverse cerebral symptoms.

Corticosteroid therapy. Prednisone is often administered to patients with fulminant hepatic failure but there is no good evidence to justify the hope that it will reduce cell necrosis.

Exchange transfusion. Coma in fulminant hepatic failure can be temporarily reversed by exchange transfusion but there is no evidence that this treatment improves final results, and some to suggest that it is ineffective.

Temporary liver support by cross circulation. This is an experimental procedure which needs further assessment.

Biochemical and haematological disturbances in fulminant hepatic failure. Abrupt loss of liver cell function in acute hepatic necrosis is often followed by biochemical and haematological and other disturbances as well as neurological abnormalities. These disturbances include: (a) Electrolyte imbalance. Hypokalaemia is the usual initial disturbance, and is followed by hyponatraemia. Acid base imbalance is also common, with respiratory alkalosis followed late by metabolic acidosis as products of tissue destruction, such as lactic acid accumulate. (b) Hypoglycaemia. This may be severe and is a direct effect of the disruption of hepatic function in carbohydrate metabolism. Frequent blood glucose determinations, and glucose infusions are needed in controlling this problem. (c) Haemostatic failure.[157] Reduced hepatic production of clotting factors can cause spontaneous bleeding. Correction by the infusion of fresh frozen plasma may be difficult because there may be a consumption coagulopathy with increased fibrinogen clearance and excessive fibrinolysis, slow heparin administration 8000 u daily, can reverse this abnormality. (d) General problems. These include increased liability to infections, and vasomotor instability with low blood pressure and oliguric renal failure.

Chronic neuropsychiatric sequelae

These include cerebral phenomena typical of hepatic encephalopathy and in addition neuromyelopathies. Spontaneous movements, reminiscent of those of hemiballismus, cerebellar incoordination, and spastic paraparesis with flexor or extensor plantar responses, and psychoses also occur.

Chronic neuropsychiatric abnormalities are particularly common after portacaval shunt procedures and vigorous attempts have been made to try and predict the likelihood of such complications, though with little success except in showing that those who have severe disease as evidenced by hypoalbuminaemia, ascites, or coma with gut bleeding are likely to do very badly.

Chapter 19

BILIARY TRACT DISEASE

GALLSTONES

Aetiology and pathology

Gallstones contain a variety of substances including cholesterol, calcium bilirubinate, apatite and crystalline calcium carbonate and mucoprotein. Bile from gallbladders with stones contains an excess of cholesterol and mucoid substances, and relatively reduced amounts of phospholipids and bile salts. Though it is not known whether these changes predispose to gallstone formation, or are induced by them, it is thought that in Western populations a reduced bile salt pool and/or excessive cholesterol secretion by the liver lead to supersaturation of bile salt solubilizing capacity and crystal deposition. In terminal ileal disease the total circulating bile acid pool (Fig. 1) is reduced, and gallstones are common.[162] Some patients with ordinary gallstones have also been found to have a bile acid pool which is half the normal size, whilst Pima Indians, who very frequently develop stones, have bile supersaturated with cholesterol.[159,161]

Pigment stones characteristic of haemolytic states are thought to represent the precipitation of non-polar unconjugated bilirubin produced by haemolysis, though it has yet to be proved to be present in bile.

The role of infection in stone formation is unclear, but at least in some people gallbladder infection is likely to initiate stone formation.

In Western communities, gallstones become commoner with increasing age, especially in obese and multiparous women, but no specific dietary or other factors predisposing to stone formation have yet been identified.[160]

Clinical features of biliary tract disease

Most gallbladders containing stones become more or less inflamed, though stones in association with ileal disease seem to be associated with curiously little reaction.

Acute cholecystitis.[164] Impaction of a stone in the neck of the gallbladder can result either in the formation of a mucocoele as the obstructed organ distends progressively, or can precipitate an acute attack of cholecystitis. Symptoms and signs then include pain and tenderness in the right upper abdomen, sometimes referred to the shoulder, fever and leucocytosis; there may also be transient jaundice and an ill-defined mass. Although acute inflammation usually subsides during or because of treatment, occasionally perforation or gangrene occur.

Biliary colic: Stones entering the duct system may pass through uneventfully, may cause symptoms of biliary colic due to intermittent obstruction, or may impact in the duct and ampulla of Vater causing jaundice or even in the ileum causing gallstone ileus (usually in the elderly).

Partial or complete obstruction of the biliary tree can result in secondary biliary cirrhosis, probably from ascending infection. The pain of biliary colic is severe and can be mistaken for that of perforated ulcer. It reaches a peak every 15 minutes, and like pain in acute cholecystitis it may be referred to the shoulder and be associated with marked abdominal tenderness and guarding. Jaundice may not be obvious at first, or at all if the stone disimpacts.

Chronic cholecystitis. Pain is seldom severe, but is usually worse after meals, especially those containing fats and clinically there is tenderness under the right costal margin especially on inspiration (Murphy's sign).

Investigation

Plain X-ray. This will show gallstones to be present in the 10 per cent of cases where they are radio-opaque. Frequent causes of confusion include renal stones, calcified lymph nodes and calcification in costal cartilages. Occasionally gas in the biliary tree will show the presence of infection with gas forming organisms (though it can also occur after biliary surgery and in gallstone ileus).

Oral cholecystography. Iodine containing contrast media will almost always delineate a normal gallbladder except in jaundiced patients, and failure of opacification usually means that there is cholecystitis with stones. Apart from stones, the examination may show a tumour encroaching on the lumen, and congenital deformity such as folding (Phrygian cap). The bile duct is seldom properly seen.

Intravenous cholangiography. Dye injected intravenously will show the extrahepatic ducts better and may show the presence of stones in a 'non-functioning' gallbaldder at oral cholecystography (due to the higher dye concentration). Failure occurs with a raised serum bilirubin (greater than 5 mg per cent). A duct with a diameter greater than 1 cm should be suspected as obstructed.

Liver function tests. These are normal in chronic cholecystitis, and a diagnosis of biliary colic or acute cholecystitis can usually be made without their aid. A raised alkaline phosphatase with a normal bilirubin are often found in incomplete biliary obstruction.

Management

Acute cholecystitis. Elective surgery. Most surgeons prefer to operate about 6 weeks after the acute episode has settled because of, or during, conservative treatment with analgesics, fluid and electrolyte replacement, and a broad spectrum antibiotic such as ampicillin; the antibiotic will not enter the obstructed gallbladder but may prevent secondary tissue invasion. The advantage of this regime is that it allows operation on a patient (who is often elderly) in the best possible physical condition, and permits diagnostic checking by cholecystography when the episode has settled.

Emergency surgery. Early (within 72 hours) operation is favoured by some surgeons who argue that it is simpler at a stage when resolving inflammation has not caused a matted mass to develop next to the liver.

If surgery is not undertaken then recurrent disease is bound to occur.

Biliary colic. The distinction of this condition from acute cholecystitis may be difficult or impossible, but treatment is similar.

Severe pain may require strong analgesics, and pethidine is

probably preferable to morphine since morphine can cause spasm of the sphincter of Oddi.

Chronic cholecystitis. It is often difficult to tell whether vague upper abdominal symptoms are really due to gallbladder disease or not. In young patients stones will in the end probably cause symptoms anyway so that cholecystectomy should be performed. In elderly patients a decision is more difficult for the operation has a distinct if small mortality rate, and the stones may never cause symptoms.

Operative cholangiography is probably a good routine procedure so that missed stones in the common duct can be detected.

Complications of gallstones and gallbladder surgery:
(a) Carcinoma of the gallbladder (see Chapter 11). This is well known to be commoner in patients with stones than would be expected by chance.
(b) Retained common duct stone and recurrent stones.
(c) Traumatic biliary duct stricture.
(d) Postcholecystectomy syndrome. Vague postprandial symptoms with fat intolerance sometimes occur after apparently successful biliary surgery. The cause is unknown.

Medical treatment for gallstones

Prolonged (several months) treatment with chenodeoxycholic acid will dissolve some gallstones completely.[163] However, it has yet to be shown to reverse any underlying cholecystitis, and it is an experimental not a clinical procedure.

EXTRAHEPATIC OBSTRUCTIVE JAUNDICE

The combination of pale stools, dark urine, high serum alkaline phosphatase and virtually normal serum transaminase is usually found (as in cholestatic hepatitis) but alkaline phosphatase levels may be completely normal. The presence of a palpable gall bladder suggests carcinoma of the head of the pancreas whilst gallstones—the usual differential diagnosis—are sometimes radio-opaque and therefore visible on plain X-ray. General causes of obstructive jaundice are listed in Table 36.

Other specialized investigations which may be necessary include hypotonic duodenography or duodenoscopy to demonstrate carcinoma of the head of the pancreas (ordinary barium meal seldom helps) and percutaneous cholangiography, on the day of operation, because of the risk of biliary peritonitis (intravenous cholangiography is not worth attempting if serum bilirubin levels are more than 5 mg per cent). Transduodenal retrograde cholangiography through a flexible fiberoptic duodenoscope is a promising procedure for expert use. Steroid administration as for instance prednisone 30 mg daily for 5 days has been shown to lower serum bilirubin concentrations in hepatocellular but not large duct obstructive jaundice but in practice does not seem a very useful test because of overlap between the two groups.

A careful investigation of a difficult case of apparent obstructive jaundice over a 3 week period is always preferable to precipitate laparotomy which will be unnecessary in cholestatic drug jaundice,[165] and dangerous in cholestatic hepatitis.

Intense itching associated with bile salt accumulation will usually respond, provided obstruction is incomplete, to treatment with cholestyramine, a bile acid binding resin. A haemorrhagic tendency due to vitamin K deficiency is common, and supplements by injection of vitamin K_1 are usually needed.

CHOLANGITIS AND BILIARY CIRRHOSIS

Inflammatory disease of the hepatic excretory system may occur as a primary or secondary condition affecting the main ducts or the intrahepatic canalicular system or both.

Table 36 Causes of obstructive jaundice

Intrahepatic
  (a) Cholestasis, drugs, pregnancy, hepatitis
  (b) Bile duct atresia
  (c) Primary biliary cirrhosis

Extrahepatic
  (a) Gallstones
  (b) Tumours of gallbladder, bile ducts and pancreas, and extrinsic compressing secondary tumours or reticulosis
  (c) Strictures, secondary to biliary surgery or inflammation and primary sclerosing lesions
  (d) Parasites, e.g. *Clonorchis sinensis*
  (e) Pancreatitis
  (f) Choledochal cyst

Primary biliary cirrhosis. This (probably) auto-immune condition is considered with other cirrhosis in Chapter 16.

Secondary biliary cirrhosis and cholangitis. Prolonged obstruction of the bile ducts, for instance due to stricture or an impacted stone is followed by periportal inflammatory change. Ultimately cirrhosis develops and is probably due to a combination of prolonged obstruction with superadded infection (secondary cholangitis).

Clinical features and treatment

Secondary cholangitis typically causes malaise, intermittent fever and fluctuating obstructive jaundice. Though usually due to gallstones or postoperative stricture it can occur with bile duct tumours or ampullary carcinoma, obstruction being temporarily relieved when tumour fragments necrose and slough. Treatment includes control of infection with antibiotics, and operation to relieve the obstruction.

PRIMARY SCLEROSING CHOLANGITIS

This rare condition of unknown cause is characterized by the presence of multiple benign strictures throughout the biliary system. The cause is unknown and there is no specific treatment.

DEVELOPMENTAL ANOMALIES

Biliary atresia. See page 121.

Choledochal cyst. This condition of congenital cystic bile duct dilation is a rare cause of obstructive jaundice, it is usually intermittent and is probably due to recurrent twisting about the cyst.

Carcinoma of the gall bladder is considered in Chapter 11.

Chapter 20

PANCREATIC DISEASE

The clinical patterns of this disease include acute pancreatitis, relapsing disease and chronic pancreatitis. All of these blend indistinguishably into each other.

Aetiology and pathology

Basic mechanisms causing pancreatitis are poorly understood; Table 37 lists the known predisposing conditions. When these are taken into account the largest group is that of idiopathic pancreatitis which can reach epidemic frequency in some areas, such as parts of southern India.

It was formerly considered that the presence of gallstones was the main factor predisposing to pancreatitis but this hypothesis is now contested because no mechanism has been clearly identified to account for such an association. Biliary reflux, such as might occur with an impacted ampullary stone, does not cause pancreatitis, except with high pressure or if there are deconjugated bile acids present (such as might occur in biliary infections) and simple pancreatic duct obstruction likewise causes atrophy rather than inflammation. It has been argued convincingly,

Table 37 Conditions predisposing to pancreatitis

Chronic alcoholism
Gallstone disease (possibly)
Familial with amino-aciduria or hyperlipaemia
With hyperparathyroidism
Secondary to hypothermia, invasive duodenal ulcer, pancreatic carcinoma, and mesenteric infarction
Mumps

however, that reflux of duodenal fluid containing active enzymic secretions will induce pancreatitis (a hypothesis that makes the operation of sphincterotomy a doubtful proposition).[166] The apparent association with gallstones may represent no more than the expected simultaneous appearance of a common disease.

ACUTE PANCREATITIS

Clinical features

Pain is usually sudden in onset, severe (occasionally equivalent to that of peritonitis) and often goes through to the back. There is marked abdominal tenderness and guarding, but usually no signs of peritoneal irritation, and bowel sounds usually remain present, if diminished. Occasionally there is mild jaundice, and sometimes peri-umbilical or flank bruising; shock, hypotension and paralytic ileus are features of severe disease.[167]

Diagnosis

A serum amylase in excess of 800 Somogyi units is diagnostic of the disease, though lower levels do not exclude it. Occasionally in doubtful cases abdominal tap with a small syringe and fine needle will yield a little fluid of high amylase content. In a few rare instances amylase circulates normally as a complexed protein (macroamylasaemia) and misleadingly high serum amylase concentrations occur.[168]

Treatment

Operation may be dangerous and has nothing to offer except diagnostic certainty in doubtful cases. Hypotension requires treatment with blood and plasma expanders since there is considerable peritoneal and tissue exudation in response to the inflammation. Oral intake is conventionally restricted to small amounts of fluids, and fluid and electrolyte balance are maintained intravenously. Drugs have little value. Pain should be treated with pethidine as morphine tends to encourage spasm of the ampulla of Vater. Anticholinergic drugs such as propantheline have the theoretical advantage of inhibiting pancreatic secretory activity but have yet to be proved clinically useful.

Controlled clinical trials have failed to show any convincing benefit from treatment with tryptic and other enzyme inhibitors, such as Trasylol.

Widespread fat necrosis can lead to calcium precipitation and tetany: parenteral calcium gluconate is then required. Diabetes may also need treatment with insulin.

Complications

Pseudocyst and abscess formation: persistent fever and leucocytosis suggest abscess formation and operative drainage may be needed. A palpable mass appearing after the acute illness is over, suggests pseudocyst formation: an accumulation of fluid in the lesser sac. Many resolve spontaneously in the course of 2–3 weeks, but drainage by marsupialization into the stomach is sometimes necessary.

ACUTE RELAPSING AND CHRONIC PANCREATITIS

Clinical features

Recurrent attacks of acute pancreatitis or continued chronic disease can cause gradual deterioration of pancreatic exocrine and endocrine function. The diagnosis of chronic pancreatitis is often difficult because pain, the dominant feature, may have no specific characteristics. Dull, boring discomfort sometimes radiating to the back may be continuous or intermittent, with no specific relieving features. Steatorrhoea due to exocrine deficiency, if present at all, is seldom conspicuous, and commonly the problem lies in differentiating from a missed peptic ulcer or psychogenic pain.

Diagnosis

In acute relapsing disease there may be a diagnostic rise in the serum amylase concentration, but none occurs in chronic pancreatitis. The presence of diabetes mellitus or more specifically pancreatic calcification on X-ray may lead to the real cause. Tests of exocrine function (secretin–pancreozymin or Lundh test) may demonstrate occult deficiency. Hypotonic duodenography may show effacement of duodenal folds due to the inflammation; pancreatic scintiscanning may show diffuse poor uptake.[170]

Treatment

This is essentially symptomatic. Analgesics (preferably non-addictive) may be needed for pain. Steatorrhoea is usually relieved by a low fat diet with pancreatic supplements.[169] Surgery may be necessary in resistant cases but there are no operations of proven value. Procedures include sphincterotomy (which has doubtful physiological validity), pancreatectomy, afferent nerve section and vagotomy with drainage. Cholecystectomy should be carried out whenever gallstones are present, despite the lack of evidence that they are aetiologically important.

ANNULAR PANCREAS

This is a rare cause of high duodenal obstruction, a ring of pancreatic tissue encircling the second part of the duodenum. It can present in infancy, or in mild cases in adult life. Treatment is by surgical bypass.

ECTOPIC PANCREAS

Rarely this is a site of acute inflammation or bleeding. It is seldom if ever diagnosed preoperatively.

FIBROCYSTIC DISEASE

Aetiology and pathology

This disease is inherited as an autosomal recessive. It is a generalized abnormality of exocrine glands, in which mucus is unusually viscid and is readily identified by the high sweat content of sodium chloride (Chapter 21).

The viscid secretions cause lung, pancreatic and sometimes liver disease by obstructing small ducts leading to proximal cystic change in the pancreas, emphysema in the lungs and periportal inflammation in the liver.

Clinical features

Infancy. In some affected babies meconium ileus occurs at birth due to difficulty in expelling the sticky secretions; occasionally there is secondary perforation.

Lung disease. The predominant problems are repeated lung infections and emphysema, and these can lead to early death.

Pancreatic disease. Steatorrhoea is seldom severe, and tends to respond well to treatment with pancreatic supplements, in the rare difficult case, medium chain triglycerides (page 47) form a useful supplement.

Liver disease. This is seldom severe or prominent.

Diagnosis

The most reliable technique employs skin iontophoresis of pilocarpine to induce sweating. The chloride concentration is greater than 70 mEq/litre.

Chapter 21

COMMONLY USED TESTS OF GASTROINTESTINAL FUNCTION

Oesophageal acid perfusion

Indication. Differential diagnosis of chest pain.

A thin e.g. 12 French gauge nasogastric tube is passed to the mid oesophagus with the patient sitting upright and coupled through a Y shaped connector and drip chambers to two bottles containing decinormal saline and hydrochloric acid. Acid is then perfused through the gullet at a rate of 5 ml per minute for 5 minutes and then if pain is not reproduced at 10 ml per minute for 10 minutes. If pain is reproduced then saline should be substituted for the acid.

Diagnostic results. Pain induced by acid and abolished by saline perfusion strongly indicates that there is active oesophagitis.

Pentagastrin test

Indications. (a) To confirm anacidity to maximal stimulation in pernicious anaemia; (b) to assess basal:peak acid output ratio in suspected Zollinger Ellison syndrome; (c) occasionally in detecting hyperchlorhydria on maximal stimulation in patients with symptoms suspected, but unproved, to be due to duodenal ulcer.

After an overnight fast a 14 to 16 French gauge radio-opaque nasogastric tube is passed into the stomach, preferably under radiological control so that it lies with the tip in the body of the stomach just to the left of the vertebral column. Resting gastric contents are aspirated, the volume noted, and discarded. With the patient lying on his left side the stomach is then aspirated by continuous suction at about 5 mmHg augmented by hand suction at 15 minutes intervals for 1 hour, this basal acid output being collected in 15 minute samples. Pentagastrin (6 μg/kg body weight) is then injected intramuscularly and the gastric secretions collected in three successive 15 minute periods.

The volume and acid concentration (with titration electrometrically to pH 7 or with phenolphthalein) are measured on all 15 minute samples and hence total output can be determined.

Diagnostic results. A pH consistently above 6·5 is diagnostic of complete gastric atrophy or the very rare achlorhydric Menetrier syndrome.

Basal to peak ratio above 40 per cent. If the total basal acid output in 1 hour is above 40 per cent of the peak acid output in the two highest consecutive 15 minute periods with pentagastrin multiplied by two (to give a similar 1-hour sampling base) then the Zollinger-Ellison syndrome is a serious diagnostic possibility.

High peak output with low basal output. If peak output is in excess of 45 mEq per hour (see above) then duodenal ulcer is a likely but not certain cause of symptoms.

Anacidity with radiological gastric ulcer. This strongly suggests gastric cancer—but is not a useful routine test, gastroscopy and biopsy being preferable.

Insulin test

Indications. The assessment of the results of vagotomy.

A nasogastric tube is passed as in the pentagastrin test positioned and resting juice aspirated. The patient then lies on his left side whilst a 1-hour (4 × 15 minute) period of basal secretion is collected by machine suction at about 5 mmHg augmented by hand suction at quarter hour intervals. Insulin (10–20 units or 0·2 units per kg body weight) is then injected intravenously and gastric secretion collected as before in 15 minute aliquots for 2–3 hours. Specimens are measured and titrated as in the pentagastrin test.

Diagnostic results. The methods of assessing positive results and their significance are disputed. A doubling in volume rate of secretion, a rise of 20 mEq per litre in concentration, or a rise of at least 1 mEq in total output over 1 hour are generally accepted criteria for positive tests. These are usually considered to represent incomplete vagotomy or re-innervation.[172]

D-xylose excretion

Indication. Indirect measurement of small bowel mucosal function in steatorrhoea.

Technique. After an overnight fast 25 g of D-xylose, a five carbon sugar, which is only poorly actively handled by the gut, is given by mouth in 500 ml of water. All urine is then collected over the next 5 hours. In patients over 50 years of age, or in whom renal disease is suspected, a serum xylose concentration should be determined at 90 minutes.

Results. Normally at least 4·5 g are excreted in 5 hours, and serum levels of at least 35 mg per cent are achieved. In idiopathic steatorrhoea this figure is reduced to less than 2·5 g (except in patients receiving a gluten free diet). Patients with Crohn's disease give results intermediate between normal values and those obtained in coeliac disease. Low values are obtained in renal disease, the elderly, and in ascitics and in gross small bowel bacterial contamination.

An alternative method employs a 5 g loading dose.

Faecal fat excretion

Chemical estimation of faecal fat excretion, whilst the patient is taking a normal mixed diet containing 70 g daily of fat, is the basic method of detecting steatorrhoea. The technique is more reliable than isotopically labelled fat uptake or loss measurements, but must be based upon a three consecutive day collection period (at least). Normal individuals excrete less than 6 g daily but patients with steatorrhoea may have variable losses which can fluctuate from apparently clearly steatorrheic to normal.

Small bowel biopsy

Indication. The investigation of malabsorptive disorders.[173]

Method. The Crosby capsule is conventionally used, it has a side port and the hollow capsule contains a cylindrical spring-loaded knife released by suction pressure which displaces a rubber membrane placed across the two halves of the capsule.

Overnight fasting is unnecessary. The capsule, preferably attached to a radio-opaque arterial catheter rather than a plain polythene tube, is placed on the back of the tongue and swallowed with sufficient tubing to reach the stomach and pass on to the duodenojejunal flexure.

Passage through the pylorus is sometimes delayed and can be aided by lying the patient on his right side and by swallowing a tablet of metoclopramide once the capsule is in the stomach. If radiology after a 2-hour interval fails to show progression then it can sometimes be achieved by passing a flexible wire guide wire down the catheter tube, thus stiffening it sufficiently to make it possible to push the tube gently through the pylorus. Once properly sited a few millilitres of saline are washed through the tube and forceful suction applied with a 20 ml syringe, thus drawing a knuckle of mucosa into the port and making a seal so that suction displaces the rubber diaphragm and activates the knife. Suction should be repeated several times to ensure firing and the capsule withdrawn.

Preliminary examination of the specimen under a low power objective or dissecting microscope may allow the characteristic flat mosaic pattern of coeliac syndrome to be identified instead of normal villous 'leaves' or 'fingers'.

Sigmoidoscopy

Indications. The investigation of rectal bleeding and other disorders of lower bowel function, and (with biopsy) diagnosis of amyloidosis and schistosomiasis.

Technique. In routine investigation no preparation is necessary or desirable for it can remove traces of blood suggesting a suprarectal lesion and can make the normal ramifying spider's web submucosal vascular pattern invisible, thus removing a valuable sign of a normal mucosa.

The thin Lloyd Davies instrument (25 cm long × 1·5 cm diameter) is usually perfectly satisfactory. The patient is placed in the left lateral position with the buttocks raised on a firm pillow over the edge of the couch, knees bent and body angled almost transversely in lordosis. After preliminary rectal examination the instrument is passed gently forwards through the anal canal in the direction of the umbilicus. As soon as the sphincter is passed the body of the instrument is manoeuvred anteriorly so that the tip now points into the sacral curve and the obturator is withdrawn. The instrument is then passed upwards under direct vision with gentle inflation as needed to see the mucosa properly. At about 15 cm from the anal verge the bowel usually turns abruptly forwards and to the left at the rectosigmoid junction. This twist can often but, not always, be negotiated by moving the hand end of the sigmoidoscope back and to the right. After full instrumentation the sigmoidoscope is withdrawn slowly to allow a second look at the mucosa.

During instrumentation any abnormalities seen can be biopsied using punch or aspiration biopsy methods.

Apart from polyps and carcinomata the main abnormalities are ulcerative lesions, either the diffuse inflammatory change of ulcerative colitis, with loss of vascular pattern, friability, easy bleeding and a deep red granular mucosal appearance with mucopus in the lumen, or more rarely discrete ulcers of amoebic dysentery. Inflammatory lesions of Crohn's disease may be distinguishable from those of colitis by the presence of granulomata in rectal biopsies in the former disease.[175]

Liver biopsy

Indications. The investigation of jaundice, hepatomegaly and generalized disease of uncertain cause and the confirmation of the presence of cirrhoses.[176]

Preliminary procedures. Prothrombin time should be within 2 seconds of the control, and the platelet count greater than 100,000 per mm^3. The patient should be blood grouped and blood should be available (but not necessarily crossmatched). The procedure should not be undertaken if the liver is unduly small (gut may be interposed between liver and parietal tissues), if the patient is unlikely to co-operate properly in breath-holding, or if there is significant anaemia, or deep jaundice (predisposing to bleeding, or to biliary peritonitis if there is extrahepatic obstruction).

Method. Premedication with a small amount of, for instance, diazepam may be needed in nervous individuals. The patient then lies on his back on a firm mattress and is supported so that his right side is at the edge of the bed and the left side is level with the right. The patient then practises a respiratory manoeuvre—taking a deep breath and then breathing out and holding his breath—so that biopsy can be undertaken in expiration. A site for biopsy is then chosen in the right midaxillary line at the site of maximal liver dullness, usually the eighth or ninth rib space (subcostal biopsy, avoiding the gallbladder, can be undertaken in gross hepatomegaly).

The site chosen is marked and after applying a skin disinfectant, sterile towels are draped around the area. Ten ml of 1 per cent lignocaine is then injected intradermally and into deeper tissues down to the pleura. A small nick is then made in the skin and the biopsy needle inserted. The choice of needle lies between the Vim Silverman, Menghini and Trucut needles. The first of these gives a better specimen in cirrhotics than the Menghini but is harder to manipulate. The Trucut also gives a good sample in cirrhotics[177] but the Menghini is easiest to handle and is probably the best used by the general operator, it consists of a wide bore needle and a small obturator which is inserted at the hub end before attachment to a fairly large (20 ml) syringe containing a few millilitres of saline. The needle is gently advanced to the pleura, identified by a respiratory 'catch' on the needle, the patient then carries out the respiratory drill and the needle is rapidly advanced, maintaining suction on the syringe, and withdrawn. The specimen usually 2 cm long may be obviously abnormal, chocolate brown in Dubin Johnson syndrome, mottled white in malignant disease, yellow if fatty, and fragmented in cirrhosis.

Complications. These are rare and include pleural and shoulder pain usually with basal collapse or a small effusion, haemorrhage, biliary peritonitis and pneumothorax.

Bromsulphthalein retention test

Indications. Diagnosis of anicteric liver disease and Dubin Johnson syndrome (see Chapter 14).

Technique. Five mg/kg body weight of dye are injected intravenously and a blood sample taken after 45 minutes. Less than 10 per cent of dye should then be retained in normal people.

Lundh test

Indication. Diagnosis of pancreatic exocrine deficiency.[178]

Technique. The tryptic content of duodenal juice is measured after a test meal of 300 ml containing corn oil (18 g), dried milk powder (15 g), glucose (40 g) and a flavouring syrup.

A radio-opaque tube size approximately 12 French gauge with a mercury loaded finger cot tip is passed into the stomach and then with the patient lying on his right side into the duodenal loop, the tip then being about 100 cm from the mouth. Duodenal juice is collected by simple siphonage into an ice cooled container during the subsequent 2 hours and an aliquot stored at $-20°C$ until estimation, when a synthetic amino-acid compound giving a colour reaction on disruption is used to measure tryptic activity.[179]

Results. Normal results are greater than 9 μEq/min/ml. Lower values suggest pancreatitis or carcinoma especially if less than 25 per cent of normal levels.

Secretin–pancreozymin test

Indication. Assessment of pancreatic exocrine deficiency.

Technique. A Dreiling double lumen tube is passed under radiological control so that the proximal limb lies in the stomach and the distal limb in the duodenal loop.

Duodenal and gastric fluid are collected separately by continuous suction and the gastric aspirate is discarded.

After a run-in period of 30 minutes 1·7 units per kg of secretin (Boots) diluted in saline is injected over 5 minutes and the duodenal fluid collected for 30 minutes (all collections being as 10 minute samples). Pancreozymin (Boots) (1·7 units/kg body weight) is then given intravenously as for secretin and the same collections are made. The volume pH, bicarbonate and lipase content of all samples are measured.

Results. Postsecretin or pancreozymin volumes of less than 50 ml, bicarbonate of less than 1·7–2·0 mEq and lipase less than 270–350 units/100 ml indicate exocrine deficiency (the first and second figures of pairs indicate results respectively with secretin and pancreozymin).[171]

BIBLIOGRAPHY

General references

1. F. A. Jones, J. W. P. Gummer & J. E. Lennard Jones, *Clinical Gastroenterology*. Oxford: Blackwell. 1968.
2. S. C. Truelove & P. C. Reynell, *Diseases of the Digestive System*. Oxford: Blackwell. 1972.
3. S. Sherlock, *Diseases of the Liver and Biliary System*. Oxford: Blackwell. 1968.
4. W. I. Card & B. Creamer (editors), *Modern Trends in Gastroenterology*, Vol. 4. London: Butterworth. 1970.
5. *Handbook of Physiology*, Section 6: *Alimentary Canal*, edited by C. F. Code. Betheda, Md.: American Physiological Society. 1967.
6. A. I. Mendeloff & J. P. Dunn, *Digestive Diseases*. Vital and Health Statistics Monographs. American Public Health Association. 1971.
7. R. B. McConnell, *The Genetics of Gastrointestinal Disorders*. Oxford University Press. 1966.
8. I. A. D. Bouchier, *Clinical Investigation of Gastrointestinal Function*. Oxford: Blackwell. 1969.

Specific references

9. F. H. Ellis, J. F. Schlegel & V. P. Lynch, Cricopharyngeal myotomy for pharyngo-esophageal diverticulum. *Annals of Surgery*. **170,** 340. 1969.
10. D. A. W. Edwards, The oesophagus. *Gut* **12,** 948. 1971.
11. F. H. Ellis, J. C. Kiser, J. F. Schlegel, R. J. Earlam, J. L. McVery & A. M. Olsen, Esophago-myomotomy for esophageal achalasia. *Annals of Surgery* **166,** 640. 1967.
12. J. R. Bennett & M. Atkinson, Oesophageal acid-perfusion in the diagnosis of precordial pain. *Lancet* ii, 1150. 1966.
13. S. Cohen & L. D. Harris, Does hiatus hernia affect the

competence of the gastroesophageal sphincter? *New England Journal of Medicine* **284,** 1053. 1971.
14. K. J. Ivey, L. Den Besten & J. A. Clifton, Effect of bile salts on ionic movement across the human gastric mucosa. *Gastroenterology* **59,** 683. 1970.
15. J. H. Baron, The clinical use of gastric function tests. *Scandinavian Journal of Gastroenterology*. Suppl. 6, 9. 1970.
16. Serum gastrin. *Lancet* ii, 1293. 1970.
17. J. E. McGuigan, Immunologic studies of gastrin. *New England Journal of Medicine* **283,** 137. 1970.
18. P. R. Salmon, P. Brown, T. Htut & A. E. Read, Endoscopic examination of the duodenal bulb: clinical evaluation of forward- and side-viewing systems. *Gut* **13,** 170. 1972.
19. R. Doll, F. A. Jones & F. Pygott, Effect of smoking on the production and maintenance of gastric and duodenal ulcer. *Lancet* i, 657. 1958.
20. R. Doll & F. Pygott, Factors influencing the rate of healing of gastric ulcers. *Lancet* i, 171. 1952.
21. R. Doll, I. D. Hill, C. Hutton & D. J. Underwood, Clinical trial of a triterpenoid liquorice compound in gastric and duodenal ulcer. *Lancet* ii, 793. 1962.
22. J. B. Cocking & J. N. MacCaig, Effect of low dosage of carbenoxolone sodium on gastric ulcer healing and acid secretion. *Gut* **10,** 219. 1969.
23. M. W. L. Gear, S. C. Truelove & R. Whitehead, Gastric ulcer and gastritis. *Gut* **12,** 639. 1971.
24. M. A. Gillies & A. Skyring, Gastric and duodenal ulcer. The association between aspirin ingestion, smoking and family history of ulcer. *Medical Journal of Australia* **2,** 280. 1969.
25. R. Doll, M. J. S. Langman & H. H. Shawdon, Treatment of gastric ulcer with carbenoxolone: antagonistic effect of spironolactone. *Gut* **9,** 47. 1968.
26. A. G. G. Turpie, J. Runcie & T. J. Thomson, Clinical trial of deglycyrrhizinized liquorice in gastric ulcer. *Gut* **10,** 299. 1969.
27. D. S. Zimmon, G. Miller, G. Cox & M. A. Tesler, Specific inhibition of gastric pepsin in the treatment of gastric ulcer. *Gastroenterology* **56,** 19. 1969.
28. H. Trevino, J. Anderson, P. G. Davey & K. S. Henley, The effect of glycopyrrolate on the course of symptomatic duodenal ulcer. *American Journal of Digestive Diseases* **12,** 983. 1967.
29. R. F. Barreras, Acid secretion after calcium carbonate in patients with duodenal ulcer. *New England Journal of Medicine* **282,** 1402. 1970.

30. M. D. Kaye, J. Rhodes, P. Beck, P. M. Sweetnam, G. T. Davies & K. T. Evans, A controlled trial of glycopyrronium and L-hyoscyamine in the long term treatment of duodenal ulcer. *Gut* **11,** 559. 1970.
31. J. E. Lennard Jones & N. Babouris, Effect of different foods on the acidity of the gastric contents in patients with duodenal ulcer. A comparison between two "therapeutic" diets and freely chosen meals. *Gut* **6,** 113. 1965.
32. J. E. Lennard Jones, J. Fletcher & D. G. Shaw, Effect of different foods on the acidity of the gastric contents in patients with duodenal ulcer. *Gut* **9,** 177. 1968.
33. J. M. Cliff & G. J. Milton-Thompson, A double-blind trial of carbenoxolone sodium capsules in the treatment of duodenal ulcer. *Gut* **11,** 167. 1970.
34. A multicentre trial. Treatment of duodenal ulcer with glycyrrhizinic-acid-reduced liquorice *British Medical Journal* **3,** 501. 1971.
35. H. Feldman & T. Gilat, A trial of deglycyrrhizinated liquorice in the treatment of duodenal ulcer. *Gut* **12,** 449. 1971.
36. H. L. Duthie, Vagotomy for gastric ulcer. *Gut* **11,** 540. 1970.
37. H. L. Duthie, K. T. H. Moore, D. Bardsley & R. G. Clark, Surgery for gastric ulcer. *British Journal of Surgery* **57,** 784. 1970.
38. J. C. Goligher, C. N. Pulvertaft, T. T. Irvin, D. Johnston, B. Walker, R. A. Hall, J. Willson-Pepper & T. Matheson, Five- to eight-year results of truncal vagotomy and pyloroplasty for duodenal ulcer. *British Medical Journal* i, 7. 1972.
39. O. Kronborg, J. Malmstrom & P. M. Christiansen, A comparison between the results of truncal and selective vagotomy in patients with duodenal ulcer. *Scandinavian Journal of Gastroenterology* **5,** 519. 1970.
40. Prevention and treatment of post-gastrectomy disorders. *Drug and Therapeutics Bulletin* **7,** 77. 1969.
41. *Postgastrectomy Nutrition*. Edited by F. Avery Jones and D. M. Krikler. London: Lloyd Luke. 1967.
42. M. J. S. Langman, Epidemiological evidence for the association of aspirin and acute gastro-intestinal bleeding. *Gut* **11,** 627. 1970.
43. Identifying the cause of gastric bleeding. *Lancet* ii, 415. 1971.
44. F. A. Jones, Problems of alimentary bleeding. *British Medical Journal* ii, 267. 1969.
45. K. F. R. Schiller, S. C. Truelove & D. G. Williams,

Haematemesis and melaena with special reference to factors influencing the outcome. *British Medical Journal* ii, 7. 1970.
46. R. F. Harvey & M. J. S. Langman, Late results of treatment for duodenal ulcer. *Quarterly Journal of Medicine* **39,** 539. 1970.
47. R. M. Donaldson, J. Hardy & S. Papper, Five year follow up study of patients with bleeding duodenal ulcer with and without surgery. *New England Journal of Medicine* **259,** 201. 1958.
48. F. C. Edwards & N. F. Coghill, Aetiological factors in chronic atrophic gastritis. *British Medical Journal* ii, 1409. 1966.
49. Intestinal absorption and its derangements. Edited by A. M. Dawson. *Journal of Clinical Pathology* **24,** suppl. 5. 1971.
50. F. A. Wilson & J. M. Dietschy, Differential diagnostic approach to clinical problems of malabsorption. *Gastroenterology* **61,** 911. 1971.
51. C. M. Anderson, Intestinal malabsorption in childhood. *Archives of Diseases of Childhood* **41,** 571. 1966.
52. T. S. Low Beer & A. E. Read, Diarrhoea: mechanisms and treatment. *Gut* **12,** 1021. 1971.
53. A. F. Hofmann, The syndrome of ileal disease and the broken enterohepatic circulation, cholerheic enteropathy. *Gastroenterology* **52,** 752. 1967.
54. S. L. Gorbach & S. Tabaqchali, Bacteria, bile and the small bowel. *Gut* **10,** 963. 1969.
55. G. M. McLeod & H. S. Wiggins, Bile-salts in small intestinal contents after ileal resection and in other malabsorption syndromes. *Lancet* i, 873. 1968.
56. B. S. Drasar, M. J. Hill & M. Shiner, The deconjugation of bile salts by human intestinal bacteria. *Lancet* i, 1237, 1966.
57. W. I. Austad, L. Lack & M. P. Tyor, Importance of bile acids and of an intact distal small intestine for fat absorption. *Gastroenterology* **52,** 638. 1967.
58. M. Shiner & J. Ballard, Antigen-antibody reactions in jejunal mucosa in childhood coeliac disease after gluten challenge. *Lancet* i, 1202. 1972.
59. P. P. Seah, L. Fry, A. V. Hoffbrand & E. J. Holborow, Tissue antibodies in dermatitis herpetiformis and adult coeliac disease. *Lancet* i, 834. 1971.
60. M. J. Kendall, S. Nutter & C. F. Hawkins, Testing gluten sensitivity by the xylose test. *Lancet* i, 667. 1972.
61. C. C. Booth, Enterocyte in coeliac disease. *British Medical Journal* **3,** 725. 1970.

62. O. D. Harris, W. T. Cooke, H. Thompson & J. A. H. Waterhouse, Malignancy in adult celiac disease and idiopathic steatorrhoea. *American Journal of Medicine* **42**, 899. 1967.
63. G. R. Plotkin & K. J. Isselbacher, Secondary disaccharidase deficiency in adult celiac disease (non-tropical sprue) and other malabsorption states. *New England Journal of Medicine* **271**, 1033. 1964.
64. W. M. Weinstein, D. R. Saunders, G. N. Tytgat & C. E. Rubin, Collagenous sprue—an unrecognized type of malabsorption. *New England Journal of Medicine* **283**, 1297. 1970.
65. M. J. Lancaster Smith, M. K. Benson & I. D. Strickland, Coeliac disease and diffuse interstitial lung disease. *Lancet* i, 473. 1971.
66. S. Shuster, A. J. Watson & J. Marks, Coeliac syndrome in dermatitis herpetiformis. *Lancet* i, 1101. 1968.
67. J. Marks & S. Shuster, Small intestinal mucosal abnormalities in various skin diseases—fact or fancy? *Gut* **11**, 281. 1970.
68. S. J. Baker, Tropical sprue. *British Medical Bulletin* **28**, 87. 1972.
69. S. L. Gorbach, R. Mitra, B. Jacobs, J. G. Banwell, B. D. Chatterjee & D. N. G. Mazumder, Bacterial contamination of the upper small bowel in tropical sprue. *Lancet* i, 74. 1969.
70. F. A. Klipstein & J. M. Falaiye, Tropical sprue in expatriates from the tropics and in the continental United States. *Medicine (Baltimore)* **48**, 475. 1969.
71. G. M. Gray, Carbohydrate digestion and absorption. *Gastroenterology* **58**, 96. 1970.
72. N. Kretchmer, Memorial lecture: Lactose and lactase—a historical perspective. *Gastroenterology* **61**, 805. 1971.
73. P. Soeparto, E. A. Stobo & J. A. Walker Smith, Role of chemical examination of the stool in diagnosis of sugar malabsorption in children. *Archives of Diseases of Childhood* **47**, 56–61. 1972.
74. J. R. Hobbs, Immunological disturbances in the pathogenesis of malabsorption. *Journal of Clinical Pathology* **24**, Suppl. 5, 146. 1971.
75. D. J. C. Shearman, D. M. Parkin & D. B. L. McClelland, The demonstration and function of antibodies in the gastrointestinal tract. *Gut* **13**, 483. 1972.
76. J. G. R. Howie, The place of appendicectomy in the

treatment of young adult patients with possible appendicitis. *Lancet* i, 1365. 1968.
77. J. Weber, N. B. Finlayson & J. B. D. Mark, Mesenteric lymphadenitis and terminal ileitis due to *Yersinia pseudotuberculosis*. *New England Journal of Medicine* **283,** 172. 1970.
78. M. D. Levitt & J. H. Bond, Volume composition and source of intestinal gas. *Gastroenterology* **59,** 921. 1970.
79. M. D. Rawson, Cathartic colon. *Lancet* i, 1121. 1966.
80. B. Smith, Effect of irritant purgatives on the myenteric plexus in man and the mouse. *Gut* **9,** 139. 1968.
81. K. W. Heaton, The importance of keeping bile salts in their place. *Gut* **10,** 857. 1969.
82. A. F. Hofmann & J. R. Poley, Cholestyramine treatment of diarrhoea associated with ileal resection. *New England Journal of Medicine* **281,** 397. 1969.
83. J. G. Banwell, N. F. Pierce, R. C. Mitra, K. L. Brigham, G. J. Caranasos, R. I. Keimowitz, D. S. Fedson, J. Thomas, S. L. Gorbach, R. B. Sack & A. Mondal, Intestinal fluid and electrolyte transport in human cholera. *Journal of Clinical Investigation* **49,** 183. 1970.
84. J. F. R. Bentley, Constipation in infants and children. *Gut* **12,** 85. 1971.
85. J. V. Verner & A. B. Morrison, Islet cell tumour and a syndrome of refractory watery diarrhoea and hypokalemia. *American Journal of Medicine* **29,** 529, 1958.
86. J. J. Bernier, J. C. Rambaud, D. Cattan & A. Prost, Diarrhoea associated with medullary carcinoma of the thyroid. *Gut* **10,** 980. 1969.
87. D. J. Holdstock, J. J. Misiewicz & S. L. Waller, Observations on the mechanism of abdominal pain. *Gut* **10,** 19. 1969.
88. S. L. Waller & J. J. Misiewicz, Prognosis in the irritable bowel syndrome. *Lancet* ii, 753, 1971.
89. H. Ellis, Colonic diverticula. Pathology and natural history. *British Medical Journal* iii, 565. 1970.
90. T. G. Parks, Natural history of diverticular disease of the colon. *British Medical Journal* iv, 639. 1969.
91. N. S. Painter & D. P. Burkitt, Diverticular disease of the colon: a deficiency disease of Western Civilisation. *British Medical Journal* ii, 450. 1971.
92. Regional enteritis. *Crohn's Disease*, edited by A. Engel and T. Larsson. Skandia International Symposia. Stockholm: Nordiska Bokhandelns Forlag. 1971.
93. J. Kyle, *Crohn's Disease*. London. Heinemann. 1972.

94. The Kveim controversy. *Lancet* ii, 750. 1971.
95. D. N. Mitchell & R. J. W. Rees, Agent transmissible from Crohn's disease tissue. *Lancet* ii, 168. 1970.
96. J. M. T. Willoughby, P. J. Kumar, J. Beckett & A. M. Dawson, Controlled trial of azathioprine in Crohn's disease. *Lancet* ii, 944. 1971.
97. J. Rhodes, D. Bainton, P. Beck & H. Campbell, Controlled trial of azathioprine in Crohn's disease. *Lancet* ii, 1273, 1971.
98. J. A. Williams, The place of surgery in Crohn's disease. *Gut* 12, 739. 1971.
99. F. T. de Dombal, I. Burton & J. C. Goligher, Recurrence of Crohn's disease after primary excisional surgery. *Gut* 12, 522. 1971.
100. J. E. Lennard Jones & G. A. Stalder, Prognosis after resection of chronic regional ileitis. *Gut* 8, 332. 1967.
101. R. Wright, Progress in gastroenterology. Ulcerative colitis. *Gastroenterology* 58, 875. 1970.
102. J. C. Goligher, F. T. de Dombal, J. McK. Watts & G. Watkinson, Ulcerative Colitis. 1968. Baillère, Tindall & Cassell.
103. S. C. Truelove, Medical management of ulcerative colitis. *British Medical Journal* i, 651. 1971.
104. J. H. Baron, A. M. Connell, T. G. Kanaghinis, J. E. Lennard Jones & F. A. Jones, Outpatient treatment of ulcerative colitis. Comparison between three doses of oral prednisone. *British Medical Journal* ii, 441. 1962.
105. A multicentre trial. Betamethasone 17-valerate and prednisolone 21-phosphate retention enemata in proctocolitis. *British Medical Journal* iii, 84. 1971.
106. J. J. Misiewicz, J. E. Lennard Jones, A. M. Connell, J. H. Baron & F. A. Jones, Controlled trial of sulphasalazine in maintenance therapy for ulcerative colitis. *Lancet* i, 185. 1965.
107. J. E. Lennard Jones, J. J. Misiewicz, A. M. Connell, J. H. Baron & F. A. Jones, Prednisone as maintenance treatment for ulcerative colitis in remission. *Lancet* i, 186. 1965.
108. F. Edwards & S. C. Truelove, The course and prognosis of ulcerative colitis: parts I and II *Gut* 4, 399. 1963; parts III and IV *Gut* 5, 1. 1964.
109. J. C. Goligher, D. C. Hoffman & F. T. de Dombal, Surgical treatment of acute attacks of ulcerative colitis, with special reference to the advantages of early operation. *British Medical Journal* iv, 703. 1970.
110. M. J. Whelton, J. M. Findlay & M. A. Macdonald,

Ileostomy and colostomy care. *British Journal of Hospital Medicine* **6**, 315. 1971.
111. D. W. Daly, The outcome of surgery for ulcerative colitis. *Annals of the Royal College of Surgeons* **42**, 38. 1968.
112. J. K. Watt, Arterial disease of the gut. *British Medical Journal* iii, 231, 1968.
113. G. E. Mavor, A. D. Lyall, K. M. R. Chrystal & M. Tsapogas, Mesenteric infarction as a vascular emergency. The clinical problems. *British Journal of Surgery* **50**, 219. 1962.
114. A. Marston, The bowel in shock. The role of mesenteric arterial disease as a cause of death in the elderly. *Lancet* ii, 365. 1962.
115. R. Doll, P. Payne & J. A. H. Waterhouse, *Cancer in Five Continents*. Berlin: Springer. 1966.
116. C. H. Collis, P. J. Cook, J. K. Foreman & J. F. Palframan, A search for nitrosamines in East African spirit samples from areas of varying oesophageal cancer frequency. *Gut* **12**, 1015. 1971.
117. I. R. Walker, R. G. Strickland, B. Ungar & I. R. Mackay, Simple atrophic gastritis and gastric carcinoma. *Gut* **12**, 906. 1971.
118. Survival tables of cancer patients registered during the years 1962–1963. *Cancer*. Sheffield Regional Hospital Board.
119. K. Engelman, W. Lovenberg & A. Sjoerdsma, Inhibition of serotoxin synthesis by para-chloro-phenyalanine in patients with the carcinoid syndrome. *New England Journal of Medicine* **277**, 1103. 1967.
120. W. S. Peart & J. I. S. Robertson, The effect of a serotonin antagonist (UML 491) in carcinoid disease. *Lancet* ii, 1172, 1961.
121. M. S. Kleinman, L. Harwell & M. D. Turner, Studies of colonic carcinoma antigens. *Gut* **12**, 1. 1971.
122. N. Zamcheck, T. L. Moore, P. Dhar & H. Kupchik, Immunologic diagnosis and prognosis of human digestive-tract cancer: carcinoembryonic antigens. *New England Journal of Medicine* **286**, 83. 1972.
123. H. J. R. Bussey, C. E. Dukes, & H. E. Lockhart Mummery, in *Cancer of the Rectum*, edited by C. E. Dukes. Edinburgh: Livingstone. 1960.
124. E. Alpert, R. Hershberg, P. H. Schur & K. J. Isselbacher, Alpha-fetoprotein in human hepatoma, improved detection in serum, and quantitative studies using a new sensitive technique. *Gastroenterology* **61**, 137. 1971.

125. H. Foy, A. Kondi, C. A. Linsell, A. M. Parker & P. Sizanet, The alpha-fetoprotein test in hepato-cellular carcinoma. *Lancet* i, 411. 1970.
126. D. M. McCarthy, P. Brown, R. N. Melmed, J. E. Agnew & I. A. D. Bouchier, ^{75}Se-seleno methionine scanning in the diagnosis of tumours of the pancreas and adjacent viscera: the use of the test and its impact on survival. *Gut* **13,** 75. 1972.
127. J. Hart, B. Modan & M. Shani, Cholelithiasis in the aetiology of gall-bladder neoplasms. *Lancet* i, 1151. 1971.
128. C. R. Sachatello, J. W. Pickren & J. T. Grace, Generalized juvenile polyposis. A hereditary syndrome. *Gastroenterology* **58,** 699. 1970.
129. I. McColl, The pathology and treatment of polyps of the colon and rectum. *Annals of the Royal College of Surgeons of England* **47,** 245. 1970.
130. A. M. O. Veale, *Intestinal Polyposis*. Cambridge University Press. 1965.
131. A. M. Ramsay, Acute infective diarrhoea. In *Diseases of the Digestive System*. British Medical Association. 1969.
132. B. Rowe, J. Taylor, K. A. Belteheim, An investigation of traveller's diarrhoea. *Lancet* i, 1. 1970.
133. R. A. Neal, Pathogenesis of amoebiasis. *Gut* **12,** 483. 1971.
134. S. J. Powell, New developments in the therapy of amoebiasis. *Gut* **11,** 967. 1970.
135. D. R. Seaton, Amoebicides. *Practitioner* **206,** 16. 1971.
136. R. A. Babb, O. C. Peck & F. G. Vescia, Giardiasis. *Journal of the American Medical Association* **217,** 1359. 1971.
137. P. Jordan, Chemotherapy of schistosomiasis. *Bulletin of the New York Academy of Medicine* **44,** 245–258. 1968.
138. H. A. K. Rowland, Intestinal schistosomiasis. *Gut* **12,** 663. 1971.
139. J. R. Anderson, in *Clinical Aspects of Immunology*, edited by P. G. H. Gell & R. R. A. Coombs. Oxford: Blackwell. 1968.
140. Clinical progress. Recent advances in jaundice. *British Medical Journal* i, 223. 1970.
141. M. Black, S. Sherlock, Treatment of Gilbert's syndrome with phenobarbitone. *Lancet* i, 1359. 1970.
142. S. Sherlock, Drugs and the liver. *British Medical Journal* i, 227. 1968.
143. A. J. Zuckerman, Serum hepatitis and the Australia antigen. *British Journal of Haematology* **19,** 1. 1970.

144. R. Wright, in *Immunology of the Liver*, edited by M. Smith & R. Williams. London: Heinemann. 1971.
145. G. C. Cook, R. Mulligan & S. Sherlock, Controlled prospective trial of corticosteroid therapy in chronic active liver disease. *Quarterly Journal of Medicine* **40,** 159. 1971.
146. A. L. Blum, R. Stutz, U. P. Haemmerli & G. F. Grody, A fortuitously controlled study of steroid therapy in acute viral hepatitis. *American Journal of Medicine* **47,** 82. 1969.
147. Alcohol and the liver. *Lancet* ii, 670. 1968.
148. M. Barry, G. Carter & S. Sherlock, Quantitative measurement of iron stores with diethylenetriamine penta-acetic acid. *Gut* **11,** 891. 1970.
149. Copenhagen study group for liver diseases. Effect of prednisone on the survival of patients with cirrhosis of the liver. *Lancet* i, 119. 1969.
150. D. V. Dhatta & S. Sherlock, Cholestyramine for long term relief of the pruritus complicating intrahepatic cholestasis. *Gastroenterology* **50,** 323. 1966.
151. The prophylactic portacaval shunt. *Lancet* i, 999. 1972.
152. K. Hourigan, S. Sherlock, P. George & S. Mindel, Elective end-to-side portacaval shunts results in 64 cases. *British Medical Journal* iv, 473. 1971.
153. R. H. Resnick, T. C. Chalmers, A. M. Ishihara, A. J. Garceau, A. D. Callow, E. M. Schimmel & E. T. O'Hara, The Boston Inter Hospital Liver Group. A controlled study of the prophylactic portacaval shunt. *American International Medicine* **70,** 675. 1969.
154. N. D. Grace, H. Muench & T. C. Chalmers, The present status of shunts for portal hypertension in cirrhosis. *Gastroenterology* **50,** 684. 1966.
155. M. H. Witte, C. L. Witte & A. G. Dumont, Physiological factors involved in the causation of cirrhotic ascites. *Gastroenterology* **61,** 742. 1971.
156. Treatment of chronic hepatic encephalopathy. *Lancet* ii, 449, 1970.
157. W. D. Walls & M. S. Losowsky, The hemostatic defect of liver disease. *Gastroenterology* **60,** 108. 1971.
158. S. G. Elkington, M. H. Floch & H. O. Conn, Lactulose in the treatment of chronic portal-systemic encephalopathy. *New England Journal of Medicine* **281,** 408. 1969.
159. Epidemiology of gall-stone disease. *Lancet* ii, 510. 1970.
160. H. Sarles, C. Chabert, Y. Pommeau, E. Save, H. Mouret & A. Gerolami, Diet and cholesterol gallstones. *American Journal of Digestive Diseases* **14,** 531. 1969.
161. I. A. D. Bouchier, Gallstone formation. *Lancet* i, 711. 1971.

162. K. W. Heaton & A. E. Read, Gall-stones in patients with disorders of the terminal ileum and disturbed bile salt metabolism. *British Medical Journal* iii, 494. 1969.
163. R. G. Dansinger, A. F. Hofmann, L. J. Schoenfield & J. L. Thistle, Dissolution of cholesterol gall stones by chenodeoxycholic acid. *New England Journal of Medicine* **286,** 1. 1972.
164. Acute cholecystitis. *Lancet* i, 428. 1967.
165. S. Sherlock, Chronic cholangitides: aetiology, diagnosis and treatment. *British Medical Journal* iii, 515. 1971.
166. K. Hansson, Experimental and clinical studies in aetiologic role of bile reflux in acute pancreatitis. *Acta clinica scandinavica* (Suppl.) **375,** 1. 1967.
167. P. A. Banks, Acute pancreatitis. *Gastroenterology* **61,** 382. 1971.
168. J. E. Berk, H. Kizu, P. Wilding & R. L. Searcy, Macro-amylasaemia: a newly recognised cause for elevated serum amylase activity. *New England Journal of Medicine* **277,** 941. 1967.
169. Today's drugs. Pancreatic extracts. *British Medical Journal* ii, 161. 1970.
170. R. N. Melmed, J. E. Agnew & I. A. D. Bouchier, The normal and abnormal pancreatic scan. *Quarterly Journal of Medicine* **37,** 607. 1968.
171. J. B. Bourke, J. C. Swann, C. L. Brown & H. D. Ritchie, Exocrine pancreatic function studies, duodenal cytology, and hypotonic duodenography in the diagnosis of surgical jaundice. *Lancet* i, 605. 1972.
172. I. S. Smith, G. Gillespie, J. B. Elder, I. E. Gillespie & A. W. Kay, Time of conversion of insulin response after vagotomy. *Gastroenterology* **62,** 912. 1972.
173. J. S. Trier, Diagnostic value of per-oral biopsy of the proximal small intestine. *New England Journal of Medicine* **285,** 1470. 1971.
174. N. Evans, L. J. Farrow, A. Harding & J. S. Stewart, New techniques for speeding small intestinal biopsy. *Gut* **11,** 88. 1970.
175. S. J. M. Goulston & V. J. McGovern, The value of rectal biopsies. *Medical Journal of Australia* i, 1234, 1972.
176. A. E. Read, Needle biopsy of the liver. *British Journal of Hospital Medicine* **5,** 84. 1971.
177. M. O. Rake, I. M. Murray Lyon, I. D. Answell & R. Williams, Improved liver biopsy needle. *Lancet* ii, 1283. 1969.
178. G. Lundh, Pancreatic exocrine function in neoplastic and

inflammatory disease: a simple and reliable new test. *Gastroenterology* **42**, 275. 1962.
179. H. S. Wiggins, Simple method for estimating trypsin. *Gut* **8**, 415. 1967.
180. L. J. H. Arthur, Juvenile pernicious anaemia. *Proceedings of the Royal Society of Medicine* **65**, 10. 1972.

INDEX

Abscess, appendicular, 56
Abscess, hepatic
　amoebic, 145
　pyogenic, 145
Abscess, subphrenic, 88
Absorption
　bile acids, 40
　fats, 41
　sugars, 49
　tests for, 175
Achalasia of the cardia, 7
Achlorhydria
　and pernicious anaemia, 34
　and ulcer, 17
Acid
　output in ulcer, 17
　output, tests of, 170
　regurgitation, 4
Acute appendicitis, 55
Adenomatous polyps, 102
Allergic gastroenteropathy, 54
Amoebiasis, 110
Amylase and pancreatitis, 166
Amyloidosis, 46
Anal canal
　congenital anomalies, 69
　fissures of, 70
Anaemia
　after gastric surgery, 28
　and malabsorption, 39
　in hiatus hernia, 4
　in liver disease, 136
　in small intestinal diverticulosis, 42
　pernicious, 34
Ancylostomiasis, 113
Argentaffinoma, 95
Ascariasis, 113
Ascites, 152
Atresia
　anal, 69
　biliary, 121
　oesophageal, 9
Atrophic gastritis, 36
Autoimmunity and
　biliary cirrhosis, 141
　pernicious anaemia, 34
　ulcerative colitis, 79

Bacillary dysentery, 106
Benign oesophageal stricture, 6
Benign tumours and polyposis, 102
Bile and gallstone formation, 159
Bile duct
　stones, 160
　tumours, 102
Bile salts
　deficiency syndromes, 40
　metabolic turnover, 41
Bile secretion and drug interference, 119
Bilharziasis (schistosomiasis), 115
Biliary
　cirrhosis, 141
　colic, 160
Bilious vomiting, 25
Biopsy
　liver, 174
　rectum, 173
　small intestine, 172
Bleeding
　colonic, 68
　upper gastrointestinal, 30
　variceal, 147
Blood groups and gastric disease, 13
Bromsulphthalein retention test, 175
Budd Chiari syndrome, 142

Cancer of
 colon, 96
 gallbladder, 102
 liver, 98
 oesophagus, 91
 pancreas, 100
 rectum, 96
 small intestine, 95
 stomach, 93
Carcinoid tumours, 95
Casoni test, 145
Chagas disease, 9
Cholecystitis, 160
Cholerrheic enteropathy, 65
Cirrhosis
 alcoholic, 134
 biliary, 141
 classification, 135
 cryptogenic, 135
Colonic functional
 disorders, 66
 ischaemia, 78
 tumours, 96
Congenital
 hyperbilirubinaemias, 121
 pyloric stenosis, 37
Constipation, 63
Crigler Najjar disease, 121
Crohn's disease
 clinical features, 74
 epidemiology, 73
 management, 75
Crohn's disease and ulcerative colitis, 77

Dermatitis herpetiformis, 44
Descending perineum syndrome, 70
Diaphragmatic herniae, 4
Diarrhoea
 functional, 64
 infective, 106
 malabsorptive, 39
 sugar, 50
Diffuse systemic sclerosis, 9, 46
Diphyllobothrium latum, 116
Disaccharide malabsorption, 50
Diverticula
 colonic, 67
 gastric, 38
 oesophageal, 2

Dubin Johnson syndrome, 122
Dumping syndrome, 26
Duodenal ulcer
 aetiology, 11
 diagnosis, 16
 gastric secretion, 17
 haematemesis and melaena, 30
 perforation, 15
 postbulbar, 16
 pyloric stenosis, 15
 treatment, 18
Dysphagia, 1

Electrolytes in gastrointestinal fluids, 62
Entamoebae, 110
Enteric fever, 107
Erosions, gastric and duodenal, 12

Fascioliasis, 114
Fat absorption and malabsorption, 42
Fat excretion, 43
Fibrocystic disease, 168
Folic acid deficiency
 in coeliac disease, 43
 in tropical sprue, 45
Food poisoning, 106

Galactosaemia, 144
Gallbladder tumours, 102
Gallstones, 159
Gardner's syndrome, 104
Gastrectomy, 25
Gastric function tests, 170
Gastric secretion
 in ulcer, 17
 in Zollinger-Ellison syndrome, 17
Gastric tumours, 93
Gastric ulcer
 aetiology, 12
 complications, 22
 medical treatment, 18
 surgical treatment, 24
Gastritis, 36
Gastroduodenoscopy, 16
Giardiasis, 112
Gilbert's disease, 121
Gluten sensitivity, 43

Haematemesis
  causes, 30
  investigation, 32
  management, 31
  prognosis, 32
Haemochromatosis, 139
Haemorrhoids, 71
Heartburn, 3
Heller's operation, 8
Helminthiasis, 113
Hepatic
  coma, 152
  scanning, 100
  tumours, 98
  vein occlusion, 142
Hepatitis
  acute, 128
  associated antigen, 129
  chronic active, 131
Hepatolenticular degeneration, 140
Hepatoma, 137
Hereditary telangiectasia, 30
Hiatus hernia, 2
Hirschsprung's disease, 69
Hookworm, 113
Hydatid disease, 145
Hydroxytryptamine, 95

Ileitis
  acute, 57
  regional, 73
Immunological deficiency syndromes, 52
Infantile pyloric stenosis, 37
Infectious hepatitis, 129
Intestinal obstruction, 58
Intussusception, 60
Irritable bowel syndrome, 66
Ischaemic
  colitis, 85
  enteritis, 57
Islet cell tumours, 101

Jaundice
  and drugs, 123
  diagnosis, 118
  haemolytic, 122
  hepatocellular, 122
  infantile, 120
  obstructive, 162

Kayser Fleischer rings, 141

Leptospirosis, 130
Liver
  abscess amoebic and pyogenic, 145
  biopsy, 174
  scanning, 126
Lymphoma of small bowel, 51

Malabsorption syndromes, 39
Mallory Weiss syndrome, 30
Meckel's diverticulum, 56
Megacolon
  aganglionic, 69
  toxic, 82
Mega-oesophagus, 9
Melaena, 30
Mesenteric
  cysts, 89
  ischaemia, 78
  lymphadenitis, 88

Non-tropical sprue, 43
Non-ulcer dyspepsia, 29

Oesophageal
  acid perfusion test, 170
  atresia, 9
  benign stricture, 6
  diffuse spasm, 8
  diverticula, 2
  reflux, 5
  sphincter, 3
  tumours, 91
  ulcer, 4
  varices, 147
  web, 6
Osteomalacia
  and gastric surgery, 28
  with malabsorption, 39
Oxyuriasis, 115

Pancreatic
  deficiency, 40
  function tests, 175
  pseudocysts, 167
  tumours, 100
Pancreatitis
  acute, 166
  aetiology, 165
  chronic, 167

Paralytic ileus, 58
Partial gastrectomy, 25
Peptic ulcer, 11
Peritoneal disorders, 87
Peritonitis, 87
Peutz Jeghers syndrome, 103
Pharyngeal pouch, 2
Pneumatosis cystoides intestinalis, 103
Polycystic liver, 145
Polyposis
  diffuse, 103
  familial, 104
  localized, 103
Portal
  hypertension, 147
  systemic encephalopathy, 155
  vein occlusion, 150
Postbulbar duodenal ulcer, 16
Postcricoid carcinoma, 92
Primary biliary cirrhosis, 141
Proctalgia fugax, 72
Progressive systemic sclerosis, 9
Protein losing enteropathy, 53
Protein malabsorption, 52
Pyloric obstruction
  adult, 37
  in carcinoma, 94
  in ulcer, 23
  infantile, 37

Rectal
  inertia, 70
  prolapse, 70
  tumours, 96
Reflux, gastro-oesophageal, 3
Regional enteritis, 73
Rotor syndrome, 122

Salmonellosis, 107
Schistosomiasis, 115
Scintiscanning
  hepatic, 126
  pancreatic, 168
Scleroderma, 9
Secretin–pancreozymin test, 176
Secretion measurement
  gastric, 170
  pancreatic, 175
Sengstaken tube, 149
Shigellosis, 106

Solitary ulcer
  caecal, 72
  rectal, 72
Splenic venography, 150
Sprue, 45
Strongyloidiasis, 116
Subphrenic abscess, 88
Sugar malabsorption, 49
Sweat test, 169

Taeniasis, 116
Tertiary contractions, 8
Trichinosis, 116
Tropical sprue, 45
Trypanosomiasis, 9
Tuberculosis
  ileocaecal, 74
  peritoneal, 154
Tumours, 91
Tylosis, 92
Typhoid, 107

Ulcer
  aetiology, 12
  duodenal, 11
  gastric, 11
  medical treatment, 18
  surgery, 24
Ulcerative colitis
  carcinoma of colon, 85
  complications, 82
  epidemiology, 78
  ileostomy, 84
  management, 80
  toxic megacolon, 82

Vagotomy, 26
Varices, 147
Vitamin B_{12} absorption, 35
Vitamin B_{12} malabsorption
  after surgery, 47
  congenital, 35
  fish tapeworm disease, 116
  pernicious anaemia, 34
  treatment, 35

Weil's disease, 130
Whipple's disease, 46
Wilson's disease, 140

Xylose excretion test, 172

Zollinger-Ellison syndrome, 14